Thank you for your purchase of *Migraine Surgery*!

Access your e-book now!

Scratch here to reveal your access code

How to redeem your code:

1. Create an account on Thieme's e-book store at ebookstore.thieme.com/register
2. Click the **My E-Books** link
3. Select **Redeem Access Code**
4. Enter this code to claim your e-book
5. You can now read your e-book online!

How to download your book for offline access:

On a compatible phone or tablet*:

1. Download the **Thieme Bookshelf** app from **iTunes** or **Google Play** after you've redeemed your access code
2. Validate your e-book store username and password
3. Select the e-book and tap to download it to your device
4. Your e-book is now available to read offline!

This app is available for iPads and Android devices. The e-book cannot be downloaded to any apps or readers other than Thieme Bookshelf.

On your PC or Mac:

1. Download **iPublishCentral Reader**** from the e-book store after you've redeemed your access code: ebookstore.thieme.com/downloadioffline
2. Validate your e-book store username and password
3. Select the book and click to download
4. Your e-book is now available to read offline!

***You may need to download and install Adobe Air prior to downloading iPublishCentral. Instructions are on the link provided.*

This code can only be redeemed one time. After redemption, it can be downloaded to multiple devices on your account. An internet connection is required for initial access and download. This book cannot be returned if the code has been revealed.

For any questions, please visit ebookstore.thieme.com/faqs.

Connect with us on social media

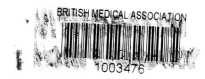

Thieme

Migraine Surgery

Bahman Guyuron, MD, FACS
Plastic Surgeon
Professor Emeritus, Plastic Surgery
Case Western Reserve University
Cleveland, Ohio

80 illustrations

Thieme
New York • Stuttgart • Delhi • Rio de Janeiro

Managing Editor: Sarah Landis
Director, Editorial Services: Mary Jo Casey
Production Editor: Torsten Scheihagen
International Production Director: Andreas Schabert
Editorial Director: Sue Hodgson
International Marketing Director: Fiona Henderson
International Sales Director: Louisa Turrell
Director of Institutional Sales: Adam Bernacki
Senior Vice President and Chief Operating Officer:
    Sarah Vanderbilt
President: Brian D. Scanlan
Printer: Replika Press Pvt. Ltd.
Illustrator: Joe Kanasz

Library of Congress Cataloging-in-Publication Data

Names: Guyuron, Bahman, author editor.
Title: Migraine surgery / Bahman Guyuron.
Description: New York : Thieme, [2018] | Includes
    bibliographical references.
Identifiers: LCCN 2018008629| ISBN 9781626236929 (print) |
    ISBN 9781626237728 (ebook)
Subjects: | MESH: Migraine Disorders—surgery
Classification: LCC RC392 | NLM WL 344 | DDC 616.8/4912—
    dc23 LC record available at https://lccn.loc.gov/2018008629

Thieme Publishers New York
333 Seventh Avenue, New York, NY 10001 USA
+1 800 782 3488, customerservice@thieme.com

Thieme Publishers Stuttgart
Rüdigerstrasse 14, 70469 Stuttgart, Germany
+49 [0]711 8931 421, customerservice@thieme.de

Thieme Publishers Delhi
A-12, Second Floor, Sector-2, Noida-201301
Uttar Pradesh, India
+91 120 45 566 00, customerservice@thieme.in

Thieme Publishers Rio de Janeiro, Thieme Publicações Ltda.
Edifício Rodolpho de Paoli, 25º andar
Av. Nilo Peçanha, 50 – Sala 2508
Rio de Janeiro 20020-906 Brasil
+55 21 3172-2297 / +55 21 3172-1896

Cover design: Thieme Publishing Group
Typesetting by DiTech Process Solutions

Printed in India by Replika Press Pvt. Ltd.   5 4 3 2 1

ISBN 978-1-62623-692-9

Also available as an e-book:
eISBN 978-1-62623-772-8

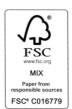

To my family for understanding my passion for the patient care, my deep desire for sharing what I know and coping with my common absence.

To the patients who suffer from this dreadful condition and helped me to discover, study, and improve the surgical treatment of migraine headaches.

Contents

Menu of Accompanying Videos

Preface

Of the discoveries that I have made, the surgical treatment of migraine headaches is the most prodigious and most gratifying one, because every time a patient tells me that I have changed her or his life it is colossally fulfilling. I have developed great respect for the patients who day after day deal with a pain level of 9 to 10. Even the mildest headache ruins one's day. Suffering from severe pain, compounded with nausea, vomiting, and light or sound sensibility is unimaginable and the reason for such a high incidence of suicide among those who are inflicted with chronic migraine headaches. These patients have the lowest level of quality of life, often become depressed, understandably, and every day search for some relief. They have no control of their lives. One of the most common and most delightful phrases that I hear from these patients is "you have given me back control of my life."

While this book offers some basic knowledge of migraine headaches, I strongly recommend making sure that every patient has the diagnosis of migraine headaches made by a neurologist. Indeed, I have never operated on a patient who was not examined by a neurologist.

This book is comprehensive and includes all the tools for successful surgical care of migraine patients who have nowhere to go. One of the most important aspects of migraine surgery is detection of the trigger sites. A successful surgery will not be attainable without this information. This book will offer means of reliably identifying the trigger site. The next needed cardinal piece of information is knowledge of anatomy. Without this information failure of the surgery is inevitable; it would be like traveling to a destination without having a map or direction. Effective surgery requires detailed technical familiarity. This book with clear illustrations and videos provides the needed information for delivering positive outcomes.

It is important to understand that while a single surgery may eliminate migraine headaches for most patients, for others surgery is a process and these patients may need more than one operation, especially those who have vague symptoms or have difficulty clearly identifying the trigger sites. Surgery on patients who are on heavy doses of opioids can be highly unpredictable. Care of these patients is also enigmatic because without relief of the pain it is hard to eliminate the dependency, and without elimination of the dependency it is difficult to judge how much of the patient's complaint is real. The decision has to be individualized. Barring this small group, dealing with the patients suffering from migraine headaches is immensely gratifying. Often, they are pleased even with some improvement although nothing short of elimination is fulfilling to me.

If just one patient were to become migraine-free as a result of the knowledge gained from this book, it would be worth all the time that I have spent developing the techniques, studying the efficacy, producing articles, giving courses, and writing this book.

Bahman Guyuron, MD

Acknowledgments

My gratitude goes to Lisa DiNardo, PhD, for her assistance in preparation of this book, and to Joe Kanasz for the masterful artwork.

Contributors

Hossein Ansari, MD, FAAN, FAHS
Neurologist/Headache Specialist
Director of Headache Clinic
Department of Neurology
University of California, San Diego (UCSD)
La Jolla, California

Bahman Guyuron, MD, FACS
Plastic Surgeon
Professor Emeritus, Plastic Surgery
Case Western Reserve University
Cleveland, Ohio

Jeffrey E. Janis, MD, FACS
Professor of Plastic Surgery, Neurosurgery,
    Neurology, and Surgery
Executive Vice Chairman, Department of Plastic
    Surgery
Chief of Plastic Surgery, University Hospitals
Ohio State University Wexner Medical Center
Columbus, Ohio

Ibrahim Khansa, MD
Clinical Instructor of Surgery
Division of Plastic and Maxillofacial Surgery
Children's Hospital Los Angeles
Los Angeles, California

Ali Totonchi, MD
Associate Professor
Case Western Reserve University
Plastic Surgery Division, MetroHealth Hospital
Cleveland, Ohio

1 History of Migraine Surgery

Bahman Guyuron

Salient Points

- Scalding of the forehead in an attempt to treat frontal migraine headaches (MHs) during the 10th century is the first ablative measure.
- Surgical attempts to mitigate MHs date back to 1923 when Jonnesco first removed the stellate ganglion.
- Walter Dandy removed the inferior cervical and first thoracic sympathetic ganglions in two patients in 1931. Dickerson described success with ligation of middle meningeal artery in 1932.
- In 1946, Rowbotham reported success with operation in three cases obtained by periarterial sympathectomy at the carotid bifurcation and excision of the superior cervical ganglion combined with ligation of the external carotid artery.
- Resection of the greater superficial petrosal nerve for the treatment of various types of unilateral headaches was suggested by Gardner et al in 1946.
- Total resection of the trigeminal nerve within the cranial base (trigeminal neurectomy) has also been tested. However, the morbidity was prohibitive.
- Murillo, in 1968, suggested removal of the temporal neurovascular bundle for treatment of MHs.
- An occipital neurectomy was suggested for patients with occipital MHs and neuritis by Murphy in 1969.
- In 1992, Maxwell reported trigeminal ganglio-rhizolysis for treatment of MHs in eight male patients through percutaneous radiofrequency.
- A retrospective study to validate the observation by patients that their headaches had disappeared after a forehead lift was completed in 2000 by Guyuron.
- The first prospective pilot study to demonstrate the role of supraorbital and supratrochlear trigger site deactivation was published by Guyuron in 2002.
- The role of single site botulinum toxin injection was report by Behmand and Guyuron in 2003.
- Dirnberger confirmed Guyuron's findings with a prospective study in 2004.
- The first randomized prospective study in surgical treatment of MHs was published in 2005 by Guyuron et al.
- Poggi also confirmed Guyuron's findings in 2008.
- The first prospective randomized migraine surgery study including sham surgery was reported in 2009 by Guyuron et al.
- The long-term efficacy of migraine surgery was documented by Guyuron's team with a 5-year follow-up study in 2011.
- For the first time, Guyuron, through a collaborative effort between three departments and using proteomic analysis and electron microscopy, demonstrated that patients who have MHs have myelin deficiency in 2014.
- The first retrospective study demonstrating the efficacy of surgical treatment in adolescent patients was completed in 2015.

1.1 Introduction

Failure of medical treatments to provide sufficient lasting and predicable relief for many patients has prompted investigators to search for a more successful solution for migraine headaches (MHs). Going back centuries ago, scalding of the frontal migraine site with a hot rod was promoted by the Andalusian-born physician Abulcasis, also called Abu El Qasim, in the 10th century. It is hard to imagine the excruciating pain and exceedingly disturbing scene related to such a primitive, drastic measure. The far-reaching nature of this approach, however, underscores the severity of the pain that migraine patients endure and how desperate they are to consent to undergo such an extreme procedure. This demonstrates one other salient fact. That is, even this far back in history, it was believed that by stopping the migraine trigger sites in the periphery one would control MH.

Surgical attempts to mitigate MH date back to 1923 when Jonnesco first removed the stellate ganglion and other parts of the sympathetic nervous system for treatment of MH. Dandy (1931), Penfield (1932), and Craig (1935) reported relief after excision of the stellate ganglion, while Love and Adson (1936) reported improvement in 12/16 patients with this technique.[1] Walter Dandy, believing that "the actual pain of MHs, so perfectly restricted to one side of the head (unless both sides are involved), must indicate an affection of nerves which carry sensation," removed the inferior cervical and first thoracic sympathetic ganglions in two patients.[2] Interestingly, he was able to eliminate MHs in both of these patients. However, this pioneer work lacked scientific significance due to a small patient sample size, absence of a control group, and an extremely short follow-up period.

Dickerson described success with ligation of the middle meningeal artery in 1932. However, Herbert Olivecrona reported failure in five of six patients who underwent ligation of the middle meningeal artery and he published discouraging results from denervation of the arteries.[3] Olivecrona also reported on tractotomy in 13 patients. Overall, 7 of 11 patients that were followed for a year had a satisfactory outcome.

In 1946, Rowbotham reported success in three cases after periarterial sympathectomy at the carotid bifurcation and excision of the superior cervical ganglion combined with ligation of the external carotid artery, which may possibly have been responsible for the success of this technique.

Resection of the greater superficial petrosal nerve in the treatment of various types of unilateral headaches was suggested by Gardner et al in 1946.[4] Twenty-six patients underwent surgery, 9 of whom were felt to have unilateral MHs, including 7 women and 2 men. All patients with MHs observed either complete elimination or significant improvement. Two patients had initial improvement, but the MHs recurred after 7 to 8 months. The authors concluded that the surgery was more successful in patients with MHs than in those with other indications. The patients, however, reported a reduction in tear production and dryness of the nose. Some patients developed corneal ulcerations. The fact that a diverse group of patients underwent the same procedure without sufficient follow-up and without controls diminishes the scientific merits of this study. Furthermore, dryness of the eyes and nose are major adverse consequences, and the former may lead to blindness, thus rendering this approach unjustifiable.

Total resection of the trigeminal nerve within the cranial base (trigeminal neurectomy) has also been advocated. Anesthesia of the ipsilateral hemiface, dryness of the cornea, corneal ulceration, and loss of vision may ensue such a complex procedure. This operation is still being performed in some centers only on patients with severe cluster-type MHs. Surgery of this magnitude is too radical and the associated morbidities are too grave. However, the effectiveness of the procedure is in accord with the contribution of a peripheral mechanism to MHs.

Murillo, in 1968, further emphasized the role of the neurovascular bundle in MH.[5] This surgery included resection of the superficial temporal artery and auriculotemporal nerve on 47 sites in 34 patients. The procedure was effective in elimination of MHs in 30 of 34 (88%) patients. This report, however, did not include the length of follow-up, nor was there a control group for this clinical trial. Wolf and his associates[6] demonstrated the role of vasomotor mechanisms in migraine-type pain in the 1940s, which supports the rationale for the surgical procedures that Murillo had suggested and those that we have devised. Additionally, Knight in 1968 suggested postauricular and auriculotemporal nerve resection for surgical treatment of MH.[7]

An occipital neurectomy was suggested for patients with occipital MHs and neuritis by Murphy in 1969.[8] This operation was performed in 30 patients. Eighteen patients had excellent results, 7 had good results, 3 had fair results, and 2 patients had poor results. Many of these patients, however, had less than a year of follow-up. Murphy's report did not indicate the incidence of anesthesia or paresthesia in the occipital region, nor did it outline any other adverse effects resulting from the surgery. Although neurectomy at this site is the last resort in our practice, it has been used in some practices as the first line of treatment by some. Nevertheless, the positive outcome of the surgery once more confirms the contribution from a peripheral mechanism in the pathogenesis of MH.

In 1992, Maxwell reported trigeminal ganglio-rhizolysis for treatment of MHs in eight male patients through percutaneous radiofrequency.[9] The patients had moderate to significant relief of MH with no reported complications. This study lacked a control group, adequate follow-up, and large enough patient sample size, similar to closure of patent foramen ovale.[10] Even techniques such as cryosurgery and injection of alcohol have been attempted for treatment of MHs. The unscientific manner in which these studies were conducted precluded any meaningful conclusions.

Statements by two patients that their MH disappeared after forehead rejuvenation at the end of 1999 prompted us to begin a study to validate this observation and the report was published in 2000.[11] After securing sufficient evidence to support what the patients reported, we designed a prospective pilot study that confirmed the role of MH surgery in 21 of 21 patients and this report was published in 2002.[12] A comprehensive study involving the four trigger sites that documented the efficacy and safety of the author's designed procedures was reported in 2005.[13] The randomized study that included a sham surgery was published in 2009.[14] In 2011, we reported the 5-year outcomes of the comprehensive study published in 2005.[15] Our study comparing the nerves of patients who did not have MH to those who suffered from MH demonstrated that the nerves in patients with MH are deficient in myelin was reported in 2014.[16]

We have demonstrated the effectiveness of peripheral trigger site deactivation on the pediatric population as well in an article that was published in 2015.[17]

References

[1] Knight G. Surgical treatment of migraine. Proc R Soc Med 1962;55:172–176
[2] Dandy WE. Treatment of hemicrania (migraine) by removal of the inferior cervical and first thoracic sympathetic ganglion. Johns Hopkins University Bulletin 1931;48:357–361
[3] Olivecrona H. Notes on the surgical treatment of migraine. Octa Med Scand 1947;128(S196):229–238
[4] Gardner WJ, Stowell A, Dutlinger R. Resection of the greater superficial petrosal nerve in the treatment of unilateral headache. J Neurosurg 1947;4(2):105–114
[5] Murillo CA. Resection of the temporal neurovascular bundle for control of migraine headache. Headache 1968;8(3):112–117
[6] Wolff HG. Headache and Other Head Pain. New York, NY: Oxford University Press;1948
[7] Knight G. Surgical treatment of migraine headaches. In: Vinken PJ, Bryn GW, eds. Vol. 5. Handbook of Clinical Neurology. Amsterdam: North Holland Publishing;1968:104–110
[8] Murphy JP. Occipital neurectomy in the treatment of headache. Results in 30 cases. Md State Med J 1969;18(6):62–66
[9] Maxwell RE. Surgical control of chronic migrainous neuralgia by trigeminal ganglio-rhizolysis. J Neurosurg 1982;57(4):459–466
[10] Morandi E, Anzola GP, Angeli S, Melzi G, Onorato E. Transcatheter closure of patent foramen ovale: a new migraine treatment? J Interv Cardiol 2003;16(1):39–42
[11] Guyuron B, Varghai A, Michelow BJ, Thomas T, Davis J. Corrugator supercilii muscle resection and migraine headaches. Plast Reconstr Surg 2000;106(2):429–434, discussion 435–437
[12] Guyuron B, Tucker T, Davis J. Surgical treatment of migraine headaches. Plast Reconstr Surg 2002;109(7):2183–2189
[13] Guyuron B, Kriegler JS, Davis J, Amini SB. Comprehensive surgical treatment of migraine headaches. Plast Reconstr Surg 2005;115(1):1–9
[14] Guyuron B, Reed D, Kriegler JS, Davis J, Pashmini N, Amini S. A placebo-controlled surgical trial of the treatment of migraine headaches. Plast Reconstr Surg 2009;124(2):461–468
[15] Guyuron B, Kriegler JS, Davis J, Amini SB. Five-year outcome of surgical treatment of migraine headaches. Plast Reconstr Surg 2011;127(2):603–608
[16] Guyuron B, Yohannes E, Miller R, Chim H, Reed D, Chance MR. Electron microscopic and proteomic comparison of terminal branches of the trigeminal nerve in patients with and without migraine headaches. Plast Reconstr Surg 2014;134(5):796e–805e
[17] Guyuron B, Lineberry K, Nahabet EH. A Retrospective Review of the Outcomes of Migraine Surgery in the Adolescent Population. Plast Reconstr Surg 2015;135(6):1700–1705

2 An Overview of Migraine Headaches

Hossein Ansari

Salient Points

- Migraine headache is the most common neurological disorder and one of the most common pain conditions, in addition to being the third most common and eight most disabling disease in the world.
- In the 2010 Global Burden of Disease Study, migraine had a global prevalence of 14.7%.
- About 11.7% of population suffer from migraine and the condition is more common in females (prevalence rate of 17.1% for females vs. 5.6% for males).
- Migraine tends to run in families and, as such, is considered a genetic disorder.
- Migraine headache incurs estimated annual costs totaling as much as $23 billion in the United States alone, including $11 billion in direct medical costs and $12 billion in lost of productivity.
- The basic physiology and underlying mechanisms contributing to the development of migraine are still poorly understood.
- While vasodilation itself may not contribute to migraine, it remains possible that vessels play a role in migraine pathophysiology in the absence of vasodilation.
- Blood vessels consist of a variety of cell types that both release and respond to numerous mediators, including growth factors, cytokines, adenosine triphosphate (ATP), and nitric oxide (NO).
- Neurons release factors such as norepinephrine and calcitonin gene–related peptide (CGRP) that act on cells native to blood vessels.
- Based on current migraine models, release of CGRP from trigeminal nerves is thought to play a central role in the painful phase of migraine due to its ability to mediate neurogenic inflammation.
- The presence of allodynia in some migraine patients, specifically chronic migraineurs, indicates that some type of "*sensitization*" take places during migraine.
- A *peripheral* mechanism with local release of inflammatory markers, which would activate trigeminal nociceptors, also probably plays an important role in this sensitization.
- Clinical presentation of the migraine can be divided into four phases including premonitory (prodromal), aura, headache, and postmonitory (resolution) phases.
- Diagnosis of migraine headaches based on ICHD-3, beta version, requires headache lasting 4 to 72 hours, and at least two of these four characteristics: *unilateral, pulsating, moderate to severe, aggravated with routine physical activity, plus one of the following: nausea and/or vomiting, photophobia*, and *phonophobia*.
- Chronic migraine (CM) is defined as headache on *15 or more* days per month, for *more than 3 months*, in which at least *8 headache days per month* fulfills the criteria for migraine described earlier.
- One important point when devising a treatment plan for the patient with chronic headache is to differentiate between *chronic migraine (CM), chronic daily headache (CDH)*, and *medication overuse headache (MOH)*.
- Neuroimaging, including magnetic resonance imaging (MRI) of the brain, is not a part of migraine diagnosis, and if the history is clear and the neurological examination is unremarkable, there is no need to perform any neuroimaging modality.
- Diagnosis and medical treatment of migraine headaches should be deferred to the neurologist treating the patients.

2.1 Introduction

Migraine is a brain disorder with attacks consisting of headache and other neurological symptoms. Nausea, vomiting, and/or sensitivity to light and noise often accompany "headache," which is the most common presenting symptoms of migraines.

The clinical course of migraine is variable over the patient's lifetime. In some patients, migraine can improve to having few or no attacks, while others might have a stable evolution and in a subset, attacks can increase in frequency over a period of time, and may become chronic.

2.2 Epidemiology and Burden

Migraine headache is the most common neurological disorder and one of the most common pain conditions, in addition to being the third most common and eighth most disabling disease in the world.[1] In the United States alone, migraine accounts for approximately 5 million primary care office visits per year.[2] In the more recent study from 2016, migraine and low back pain were the leading causes of Years Lived with Disability (YLDs) in high-income, high-middle-income, and middle-socio-demographic Index countries.[3] In the 2010 Global Burden of Disease Study, migraine had a global prevalence of 14.7%.[4]

In childhood, it is slightly predominant in males, but after puberty, a 3:1 female predominance is established. Ninety percent of migraine patients have their first attack by the age of 40 years. In the United States, it is estimated that 11.7% of population suffer from migraine and the condition is more common in females (prevalence rate of 17.1% for females vs. 5.6% for males).[5] Migraine tends to run in families and, as such, is considered a genetic disorder.

Migraine is a common public health and socioeconomic burden worldwide. It can negatively affect quality of life and productivity both at work and at home[6] and is often underdiagnosed or misdiagnosed and undertreated or mistreated.[7–9] Migraine headache incurs estimated annual costs totaling as much as $23 billion in the United States alone, including $11 billion in direct medical costs and $12 billion in lost of productivity.[10,11]

Despite its prevalence, the basic physiology and underlying mechanisms contributing to the development of migraine are still poorly understood and the development of new therapeutic targets is long overdue.

2.3 Pathophysiology

In 1938, Wolff and Graham suggested that the head pain of the migraine attack is produced by distension of the cranial arteries. In 1963, Wolff hypothesized the vascular theory of migraine, which for many years was accepted as the pathophysiology of migraine until the trigeminocervical (trigeminovascular) theory of migraine replaced the vascular theory. Based on this theory, activation of trigeminovascular afferents in the meninges releases *inflammatory neuropeptides* and other small molecules that promote neurogenic inflammation and development of *peripheral sensitization* of the primary nociceptive neurons. The trigeminovascular pathway conveys nociceptive information from the meninges to the brain. The pathway originates in trigeminal ganglion neurons, whose peripheral axons reaches the pia, dura, and large cerebral arteries,[12] and its central axons reach the nociceptive dorsal horn laminae of the spinal nucleus V.[13]

The role of vasodilation in migraine is unclear and recent findings challenge its necessity. While vasodilation itself may not contribute to migraine, it remains possible that vessels play a role in migraine pathophysiology in the absence of vasodilation. Blood vessels consist of a variety of cell types that both release and respond to numerous mediators, including *growth factors*, *cytokines*, *adenosine triphosphate (ATP)*, and *nitric oxide (NO)*. Many of these mediators have actions on neurons that can contribute to migraine. Conversely, neurons release factors such as *norepinephrine* and *calcitonin gene–related peptide (CGRP)* that act on cells native to blood vessels. Both normal and pathological events occurring within and between vascular cells could thus mediate bidirectional communication between vessels and the nervous system, without the need for changes in the vascular tone. CGRP has been strongly linked to migraine pathology. Based on current migraine models, release of CGRP from trigeminal nerves is thought to play a central role in the painful phase of migraine due to its ability to mediate neurogenic inflammation.[14]

Unlike other pain states, migraine sufferers report multiple distinct triggers. These triggers are innocuous in healthy patients, which suggest that the sensitivity to different triggers in migraine is due to maladaptive changes within the nervous system. The presence of allodynia in some migraine patients, specifically chronic migraineurs, indicates that some type of "*sensitization*" takes place during migraine. Although it is clear that *central* pathology is the main reason for this phenomenon, a *peripheral* mechanism with local release of inflammatory markers, which would activate trigeminal nociceptors, also probably plays an important role in this sensitization.[15] The key to understanding the pathophysiology of migraine is the concept of *peripheral and central sensitization* of trigeminal nociceptive neurons.[14]

In many cases, migraine attacks are likely to begin centrally, in brain areas capable of generating the classical neurological symptoms of prodromes or aura, whereas the headache phase begins with consequential activation of meningeal nociceptors at the origin of the trigeminovascular system.

In summary, the extent of these diverse symptoms suggests that migraine is more than a *headache*. It affects multiple cortical, subcortical, and brainstem areas that regulate autonomic, affective, cognitive, and sensory functions. Therefore, migraine is viewed as a complex, neurological disorder with a strong genetic component; *headache* is the most common presenting symptom of this complex condition. There is currently no objective diagnosis or treatment (cure) that is universally effective in aborting or preventing attacks.

2.4 Clinical Presentation

As discussed in the Pathophysiology section, migraine is not merely a headache, but a complex neurological disorder. Clinical presentation of the migraine can be divided into the following *four phases*[16-18]:

- **Premonitory phase (prodromal):** Symptoms that precede the other symptoms of the migraine attack by 2 to 48 hours and forewarn of other symptoms to come. Symptoms of this phase include a range of nonspecific complaints such as food cravings, yawning, irritability, unhappiness, euphoria, somnolence, hyperactivity, difficulty concentrating, bloating, fatigue, stiff neck, insomnia, anxiety, and so on.

  Due to the nonspecific nature of these complaints, most patients do not consider them as being part of the migraine and do not report them, unless specifically asked by the physician.

- **Aura phase:** About 25 to 30 % of patients with migraine report *transient focal neurological* symptoms, which are known as aura. Migraine with aura is referred to as "classic migraine" as opposed to migraine without aura, which is known as "common migraine." The most common type of aura is *visual aura*, which can present as the following:
  - A shimmering arc of white or colored lights, followed by a blind spot or peripheral vision loss (scintillating scotoma).
  - A zigzag appearance of lines in the visual field (fortification spectra).
  - A change in the perception of the shape of viewed objects (metamorphopsia).

Other types of *aura* include the following:
  - *Sensory aura:* a feeling of numbness (paresthesia), mostly unilateral, which is most common

in the face (involving the tongue) and hand (chiro-oral pattern).
  - *Language/speech aura:* presents with slurred speech, difficulty finding words or frank dysphagia.
  - *Motor aura:* relatively rare type of aura, which presents with objective weakness of limb muscles, usually occurring unilaterally. This type of aura is mostly seen in a certain type of migraine referred to as hemiplegic migraine, which has known genetic etiology.
  - *Brainstem aura:* presents with at least two of the following symptoms:
    - Dysarthria (speech difficulty).
    - Vertigo (feeling of room spinning).
    - Tinnitus (ear ringing).
    - Hypacusis (impairment of hearing).
    - Diplopia (double vision).
    - Ataxia.
    - Decreased level of consciousness.
  - *Retinal aura:* similar to visual aura, but occurs in only one eye. This type of aura is very rare.

Each individual aura symptom lasts *5 to 60 minutes* and the aura is accompanied with or is followed by a headache *within 60 minutes*, although some individuals experience aura without headache, which is referred to and known as "migraine equivalent." Conversely, aura does not necessarily accompany each migraine attack in patients who have migraine with aura.

- **Headache phase:** This is the painful phase of migraine, which catches the attention of most patients, prompting them to seek medical attention. The typical migraine headache *starts unilaterally and* has a throbbing (pulsating) quality. It can be associated with nausea, vomiting, and/or sensitivity to light, noise, and smell. The area of the head or neck where the headache phase starts is usually referred to as a **trigger point**. The location of the trigger points is extremely important when planning the treatment strategy for each individual patient.

  Migraine pain can also be accompanied by abnormal skin sensitivity (allodynia) and muscle tenderness. The headache of the migraine ranges from moderate to severe and although it usually starts on one side of the head, it can later spread to involve the entire head. Also, it is not uncommon for the headache to start from more than one area at the same time. The duration of headache phase of migraine is between *4 and 72 hours*. If the duration of headache attack lasts more than 72 hours (without remitting), it is classified as "*status migrainosus*."

  As the headache progresses, it may be accompanied by a variety of autonomic symptoms (nausea, vomiting, nasal congestion, rhinorrhea, lacrimation, ptosis, yawning, frequent urination, and diarrhea), affective symptoms (depression and irritability), cognitive symptoms (attention deficit, difficulty finding words, transient amnesia, and reduced ability to navigate in familiar environments), and sensory symptoms (photophobia, phonophobia, osmophobia, muscle tenderness, and cutaneous allodynia).[17]

• **Postdrome (resolution) phase:** This is the period after the headache phase has ended and is associated with fatigue, irritability, concentration difficulty, and other nonspecific complaints.

A summary of the four phases is shown in ▶ Fig. 2.1.

In order to standardized the diagnosis of headache disorders, including migraine, the International Headache Society (IHS) developed the classification, entitled the International Classification of Headache Disorders (ICHD), the first version of which was published in 1988. Since then, multiple revisions have been made in this classification and the latest edition (*ICHD-3, beta version*) was released in 2013.[19] The ICHD provides explicit operation diagnostic rules and a common language facilitating communication on a global level.

ICHD-3, beta version, classifies migraine as follows:

At least FIVE Headache attacks, each lasting **4 to 72 hours** and fulfilling criteria A and B below:

A. Headache with at least TWO of the four characteristics:
   1. Location: unilateral.
   2. Quality: Pulsating.
   3. Intensity: moderate to severe.
   4. Aggravation: by routine physical activities.
B. During headache, at least one of the following two features is present:
   1. Nauseas **and/or** vomiting.
   2. Photophobia **and** phonophobia.

As evident, this classification and criteria are very clear and simple. This classification is available online and is easy to use by all specialties. Using these criteria can be very helpful in standardizing the diagnosis of migraine and avoiding its misdiagnosis with other headache disorders.

There are certain known triggers for migraine. Common triggers are stress, sleep disturbance, dehydration, missing a meal (fasting), alcohol (especially red wine), weather and barometric pressure changes, flickering lights, and menstrual cycles. Also certain foods such as monosodium glutamate (MSG) or nitrate containing foods, artificial sweeteners (like diet sodas) and certain smells like strong perfumes, smoke, and cleaning chemicals can trigger headache attacks in patients with migraine.

2.5 Chronic Migraine

Based on ICHD-3, beta version, CM is defined as headache on *15 or more* days per month, for *more than 3 months*, in which headache of at least *8 of the 15 headaches* fulfills the criteria for migraine[19] described earlier.

CM is a debilitating condition affecting approximately 2% of the general population.[20] CM is associated with significant disability and reduced health-related quality of life.[21,22] CM usually remains underdiagnosed and is poorly treated. In addition, treatment options are limited.

One important point when devising a treatment plan for the patient with CM is to differentiate between CM, Chronic Daily Headache (CDH), and Medication Overuse Headache (MOH). CDH is a descriptive term that encompasses several different specific headache diagnoses, including migraine, tension-type headache, cluster headache, or any other headache disorder.

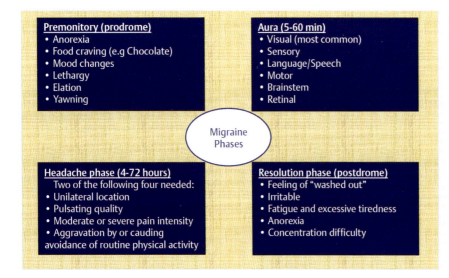

Fig. 2.1 Four clinical phases of migraine syndrome.

MOH, which is also known as "rebound headache," is a secondary headache disorder that frequently complicates the management of multiple primary headache disorders. Based on ICHD-3, beta version, MOH is defined as headache occurring on 15 or more days per month developing as a consequence of regular overuse of acute or symptomatic headache medication (on 10 or more, or 15 or more days per month, depending on the medication) for more than 3 months.[19]

This is very important, since in practice, most patients suffering from CDH in reality have a combination of migraine and MOH. Therefore, this is very important when planning the treatment strategy, since most of the time the management of the MOH will in turn reduce the underlying migraine frequency and increase response to treatment.

2.6 Determination of Trigger Points in Patients with Migraine Headache

As discussed in the previous section Clinical Presentation, the area and pattern in which the headache initiates are crucial in determining the trigger point of the headache phase in patients with migraine.

A detailed history plus a thorough head and neck examination is often sufficient to determine the trigger point(s) in migraine patients. A few helpful keys are as follows:

- Patients who complain of headaches, which start from the back of the eye(s), back of the nose, or from the maxillary sinus area, usually have an *intranasal trigger point(s)*. This could be due to a severe septal deviation with contact to the lateral nasal wall, septal spur, or concha bullosa. These patients tend to wake up with headache, and their headaches are usually correlated with weather, especially barometric pressure changes. These patients are commonly mislabeled as having *sinus headache* and as such, frequently treated with unnecessary antibiotics. The presence of autonomic features (watery eye or nasal congestion) in about 10 to 20% of migraineurs also contributes to the common misdiagnosis of their condition as *sinus headache*.
- Patients who complain of pain above the eyebrows usually have supraorbital or supratrochlear (or both) nerve irritation, mostly due to pressure from corrugator supercilii muscles. These patients usually have deep frown lines (especially if they are longtime migraineurs) due to corrugator muscle hyperactivity. These patients also often report that the use of a hot or cold compress or even putting pressure on the area above the eyebrow with their fingertips helps their headache.

- Patients who report their headaches start from the side of the head usually have irritation of either the *zygomaticotemporal nerve* (*ZTN*) or the *auriculotemporal nerve* (*ATN*), both of which are small branches of the trigeminal nerve.
  - Patients with ATN irritation usually show the area of the pain to be superficially right at the area where the hairline starts. These patients tend to use hot or cold compresses on the area and sometimes experience tenderness of the scalp, for example, when combing their hair.
  - Patients with ZTN trigger, on the other hand, complain of more deep pain in the temporal area. They usually have tenderness of the masseter muscles, and if the duration of the headache is long, sometimes hypertrophy of muscles is prominent. Using a hot or cold compress usually does not help alleviate the pain in these patients, since ZTN is deep in the muscle. These patients are commonly diagnosed as having temporomandibular joint dysfunction and often undergo unnecessary treatment, including the prescription of a mouth device or even surgical intervention. A detailed examination by an experienced physician or dentist is required in order to distinguish these patients from those with bruxism or TMJ dysfunction as the potential migraine trigger. Also, a detailed examination and identification of the anatomic location of the pain by digital tenderness can often distinguish between ATN and ZTN triggers, although it is not uncommon for a patient to have both trigger sites.
- Patients with *occipital trigger point*(s) usually complain of headaches, which start at the back of the head, neck, or sometimes even the shoulder area. Patients describe deep pain in the area, which then radiates to the temporal, parietal, vertex, or even frontal region. These patients usually cannot tolerate any physical activity, since it rapidly triggers the headache. In examination, tightness of cervical paraspinal and trapezius muscles is usually prominent and the anatomic landmark of the greater and lesser occipital nerves has severe digital tenderness. These patients usually report changing their pillow to help improve the headache without any success. Also, they often seek treatment from chiropractors, which sometimes worsens the headache, because manipulation can further irritate the occipital nerve(s). These patients have a relatively good response to occipital nerve blocks and it is not uncommon for them to undergo unnecessary procedures, including nerve ablation or stimulators, which are often unhelpful and may even worsen the migraine. The most common misdiagnoses of the occipital migraine (which is sometimes called *cervicogenic migraine*) are occipital neuralgia (*ICHD-3,*

section 13.4) and cervicogenic headache (*ICHD-3, section 11.2.1*).

By utilizing the ICHD-3 guidelines, it is easy to differentiate between occipital neuralgia and migraine. Neuralgia, which is defined as paroxysmal attacks lasting from a few seconds to minutes, is totally different than migraine headache, which is a throbbing pain lasting more than 4 hours. However, in practice, migraine patients with occipital trigger point are sometimes misdiagnosed as occipital neuralgia just based on the location of the pain.

On the other hand, there is some overlap between migraine and cervicogenic headache in ICHD-3, which can sometimes make the differential somewhat challenging.

In summary, migraines with occipital trigger(s) can be clearly distinguished from the other two headache conditions by using ICHD-3 in combination with a detailed history and head/neck examination; however, in practice, the ICHD-3 criteria are underutilized. This results in the misdiagnosis of migraine and its mistreatment as occipital neuralgia or cervicogenic headache.

2.7 Imaging in Patients with Migraine

Neuroimaging, including magnetic resonance imaging (MRI) of the brain, is not a part of migraine diagnosis; if the history is clear and the neurological examination is unremarkable, there is no need to perform any neuroimaging modality. In fact, performing a computed tomography (CT) scan or MRI of the brain in patients with migraine often creates unnecessary worry due to incidental finding(s), and this in turn makes headache management more difficult. Common incidental findings that can be seen with advanced imaging include the following:
• Pituitary lesion (cyst, hyper or hypodense lesion).
• Partially empty sella.
• Colloid cyst.
• Arachnoid cyst.
• Pineal cysts.
• Nonspecific T2 finding, which is sometimes reported as a demyelination lesion by inexperienced radiologists.
• Low-lying cerebral tonsils, which can be reported as a Chiari malformation.
• Vascular anomalies such as venous angioma, capillary telangiectasia, small aneurysms.

It is sometimes very difficult to convince patients who are reported to have any of the above findings that these findings do not have any clinical significance. A more unfortunate result of these advanced imaging studies is that some patients go on to undergo unnecessary brain surgery for some of the above incidental findings, which often makes headache control extremely difficult.

On the other hand, in patients whose history and examination is suggestive of an intranasal trigger point, a CT scan of the nose and paranasal sinuses may provide valuable information, which can aid in developing an appropriate treatment plan.

In summary, besides obtaining a comprehensive history, which is the key for diagnosing headache disorder, a very detailed head, neck, and nose examination should be part of the initial consultation in headache patients.

2.8 Treatment

Treatment of migraine includes abortive (acute, as needed) and preventive (prophylactic, daily) options.

2.8.1 Abortive Treatment

All migraine patients require abortive therapy to stop the migraine attack. Without abortive treatment, migraine attacks cause significant disability. Based on a World Health Organization (WHO) report, migraine ranked eighth among all disorders causing years of life lived with disability.[23]

Attention to the following considerations will increase the effectiveness of abortive treatment:
• *Treat the attack early*: Unlike other pain disorders, when administering abortive therapy to migraine headaches, it is always recommended that the patient take the medication early in the attack for increased benefit. This standard is commonly not adhered to by patients, who often think they need to tolerate the headache until it becomes severe enough to warrant taking abortive treatment. All abortive migraine treatments tend to be more effective if taken early in the headache attack.
• Some patients might require more than one class of migraine abortive therapy.
• Proper route of administration of migraine abortive treatment must be considered in individual patients. For example, migraine patients who develop severe nausea and vomiting during their attacks will require nonoral medication.
• More importantly, the use of abortive therapy should be limited based on the class of medication that can be used in order to avoid development of MOH. This is especially important when patients use over-the-counter medication where there is no limitation or control on the amount they may use within any given period of time.

Patients often underestimate the amount of the over-the-counter medication used. For this reason, we always prefer patients to have prescription abortive therapy in order to control the amount of the medication taken. The limitation of use in each abortive class will be discussed in the individual class section below.

The following five main classes of abortive (acute) therapies are standard treatment for migraine headache:

• **Simple analgesics:** These are usually the first-line agents and most patients use this class of therapy even prior to seeking medical attention. The key in using this class of medication is proper dosage. Simple analgesics are divided into two categories:
  - *Acetaminophen:* this is probably the safest class of migraine abortive treatment, but is also likely to be the least effective. The dose per attack is 1,000 mg with a maximum daily dose of 3,000 mg. In terms of its limitations, acetaminophen can be used up to 15 to 20 days per month.
  - *Nonsteroidal anti-inflammatory drugs (NSAIDs):* this class is probably the most commonly used over-the-counter migraine abortive therapy. The most commonly used drugs in this class are as the following:
    ○ *Ibuprofen:* The dose per attack is 400 to 800 mg and a maximum daily dose of 2,400 mg/d. A solubilized form of ibuprofen in the liquid-containing capsules is probably slightly more effective, since it has faster onset of action.
    ○ *Naproxen sodium:* The dose per attack is 500 to 550 mg with a maximum daily dose of 1,375 mg/d. The benefit of naproxen versus ibuprofen is a longer half-life (14 hours compared to 2 hours) and a downside is its slower onset of action.
    ○ *Diclofenac:* In the form of *potassium* salt, it is probably the most effective NSAID for migraine attacks, since it has a rapid onset of action and shorter maximal plasma concentration. Dose is 50 mg per attack with a maximum daily dose of 150 mg/d. There are different tablet and capsule formulations of diclofenac potassium and also a powder for an oral solution (all formulations are 50 mg), the latter of which is the only FDA (Food and Drug Administration) approved NSAID for the acute treatment of migraine.[24]

In summary, NSAIDs are a commonly used and relatively effective migraine abortive agent, since they can be administered in pill form (diclofenac potassium, ibuprofen, naproxen sodium), by injection (such as ketorolac), dissolved in water, (diclofenac potassium for oral solution), suppository (rectal Indomethacin), or via nasal spray (nasal ketorolac). Major side effects of the long-term use of NSAIDS are nephrotoxicity and gastrointestinal (GI) adverse effects including peptic ulcer. In terms of limitations, in order to avoid MOH, NSAIDS can be used up to 15 to 20 days per month.

• **Triptans:** This class of medication is referred to as the gold standard abortive therapy for migraine and these are selective agonists of *serotonin receptors* (5HT-1), subtypes B and D. They were introduced to the market in 1992 and despite being the most effective drugs for acute treatment of migraine,[25] they are still underutilized. Currently *seven triptan* agents are available in the United States, which, based on their half-life, can be divided into three categories:
  - Short acting: sumatriptan, rizatriptan, zolmitriptan, almotriptan, and eletriptan.
  - Intermediate acting: naratriptan.
  - Long acting: frovatriptan.

All seven triptan drugs are available in tablet form, and some are also available in other formulations.

Sumatriptan is the prototype and oldest triptan and has the most variety in terms of formulations. In addition to its tablet form, it is available as a nasal spray, various subcutaneous injections, and the novel formulation of nasal powder delivered by a breath powder delivery device.[26]

Potential adverse effects of triptans, which are mainly secondary to smooth muscle vasoconstriction, include pressure and tightness of the chest and throat, a flushing sensation, and paresthesia. These adverse effects are sometimes referred to as "triptan sensation."

Major contraindications for the use of triptan are cerebrovascular disease, coronary artery disease, peripheral vascular disease, uncontrolled hypertension, and severe liver disease.

In terms of limitations (to avoid MOH), triptans can be used up to 9 to 10 days per month. In summary, triptans are the most effective drugs for acute migraines and are considered the gold standard therapy in migraine.

• **Ergot agents:** Ergot alkaloids have been used for many years for migraine. Although oral ergotamine tartrate is difficult to obtain in the United States, nasal sprays and injectable formulations of ergotamine in the form of dihydroergotamine mesylate are commonly used by headache experts for the acute therapy of migraine. Specifically, intravenous (IV) injection/infusion of dihydroergotamine mesylate in the form of *D.H.E. 45* is one the best therapies for patients with status migrainosus.

Major adverse events are GI symptoms (nausea, abdominal cramps), acroparesthesia, chest tightness, and leg cramps. In addition to all the contraindication of triptans (see above), this class of medication is contraindicated during pregnancy.

- **Isometheptene-containing agents:** These agents provide a combination of isometheptene with acetaminophen and dichloralphenazone, and are one the oldest abortive therapies for migraine. Isometheptene is sometimes better tolerated than triptans. Major contraindications are coronary artery disease and ischemic stroke.
- **Caffeine-containing analgesics:** There are four formulations of caffeinated analgesics used for the abortive treatment of migraine:
  - Combination of 500-mg acetaminophen and 65-mg caffeine: available over the counter.
  - Combination of 250-mg acetaminophen, 250-mg aspirin, and 65-mg caffeine: available over the counter.
  - Combination of ergotamine with caffeine (1 mg/100 mg): a prescription medication, which has the highest amount of caffeine.
  - Combination of acetaminophen/caffeine/ isometheptene (325 mg/20 mg/65 mg): a prescription drug that has the lowest amount of caffeine in this class of medication.

There is a combination of caffeinated *butalbital*-containing agents: available in the US market and although sometimes prescribed for the abortive treatment of migraine, these agents have never been approved for migraine treatment. Due to its very high potential for dependence and the development of medication overuse (rebound) headache plus reports of serious adverse events, including death from sudden withdrawal, use of this class of medication is not recommended in patients with migraine under any circumstance.[27-29]

The main issue with the use of caffeinated medication is the development of MOH with the excessive use of caffeine. This is especially relevant when the patient takes the over-the-counter formulation, in which case it is difficult to control the number of days that patients use this medication. In practice, a majority of patients who are seen in tertiary headache clinics and use the over-the-counter caffeinated analgesics develop MOHs. For this reason, we usually do not recommend this class of medication as a common treatment for migraine.

Other classes of medication that can sometimes be used as migraine abortive (acute) agents are the following[30]:

- Anti-dopaminergic antiemetic agents, especially prochlorperazine and metoclopramide, which are mainly used as adjunctive therapy with NSAIDs or triptans in patients with migraine. IV administration of these agents is part of protocol for migraine patients who present to emergency departments.
- Steroid: both oral and IV administrations are used frequently in patients with migraine.
- Valproate sodium: IV administration of this antiepileptic agent is shown to be effective for acute treatment of migraine in some small studies.
- Magnesium: IV administration of magnesium sulfate has been used with varied results in patients with migraine.
- Opioid analgesics: due to high risk of dependency and the potential for development of MOH, the use of this class of medication should be limited to patients who have clear contraindication or lack of response to **all** of the above five classes of abortive treatment. In general, we do not recommend using opioid in patients with migraine. If this class is to be used, a limitation of a maximum of 5 days per month needs to be considered in order to decrease the chance of MOH.

2.8.2 Preventive Treatment

Based on headache frequency, some percentages of migraine patients also require preventive therapy to reduce the frequency (and sometimes even intensity) of migraine attacks. Preventive treatment is used to reduce the frequency, duration, or severity of migraine attacks.

Also using preventive therapy might enhance the response to abortive treatment, improve patient's ability to function, reduce disability related to headache,[31] and finally reduce health care costs.[32]

A preventive migraine medication is considered successful if it reduces migraine attack, frequency, or headache days by at least 50% within 3 months. Studies show that preventive migraine medication is underutilized and only 13% of all patients with migraine currently use preventive treatment.[33]

Three main classes of medication commonly used for migraine prevention are the following:

- **Antidepressants:** Tricyclic antidepressants (mainly amitriptyline and nortriptyline) and serotonin-norepinephrine reuptake inhibitors (mainly venlafaxine) are the mostly used drugs in this class.
- **Antihypertensive:** Beta-blockers (especially propranolol, nadolol, and timolol), calcium channel blockers (verapamil, flunarizine), and more recently angiotensin receptor antagonists (candesartan) are the most commonly used drugs in this class.
- **Antiepileptics:** Topiramate, divalproex sodium, and gabapentin are the most commonly used medications in this class.

Other agents and medications sometimes used as preventive treatment include herbal medication (e.g., *Petasites*), natural supplements (magnesium), and vitamins (riboflavin).

The key in using preventive treatments is slow titration and using the correct (target) dose of drug.

A major limitation in using preventive therapy is the development of adverse events plus the possibility of drug interaction.[34] Due to these limitations, non-pharmacological (*procedural*) treatment for migraine has always been a popular treatment commonly used for patients with migraine. The most common procedural treatments of migraine are discussed below.

Onabotulinum toxin A Injection

Onabotulinum toxin A (BT-A) has been and is still used for the treatment of different types of headache disorder. However, after two large multicenter studies called PREEMPT (the Phase III Research Evaluating Migraine Prophylaxis Therapy) trials,[35,36] its use was FDA approved for the treatment of chronic migraine.

BT-A injects intramuscularly in different muscle groups.

Three methods of injection commonly used for BT-A are as follows:
- **Fixed-site, fixed-dose method**: this method uses symmetrical injection sites and a range of predetermined doses, where 155 units of BT-A is administered at 31 injections sites across seven specific head and neck muscle groups as shown in ▶ Table 2.1.
- **Follow-the-pain method**: often employs asymmetrical injections and adjusts the sites and doses depending on where the patient feels pain and where the examiner can elicit pain and tenderness on palpation of the muscles.
- **Combination method**: uses injections at fixed sites with fix dose, supplemented with follow-the-pain injection(s).

Peripheral Nerve Block

Peripheral nerve blocks (PNBs) are one of the most widely accepted interventional treatment of differ-ent type of headaches including migraine.[37] Different peripheral nerves can be targeted based on patient symptomatology. The most common nerves that are blocked in migraine headache are the greater occipital, lesser occipital, auriculotemporal, zygomaticotemporal, supraorbital, and supratrochlear nerves. Less commonly, the posterior auricular and third occipital also can be targeted. Blockage is performed using local anesthetic (lidocaine, bupivacaine). Some physicians add steroid to local anesthetic with the assumption that it might increase the duration of block; however, adding steroid to local anesthetic, at least in migraine patients, has not been shown to be effective.[38]

Neuromodulation

Different neuromodulation devices have been used, and some are under study or under development for treatment of primary headache disorders, which we are sure to hear more about in the future.

Here, we mention some of the most commonly used neuromodulation devices[39]:
- Pericranial peripheral nerve stimulation: The Cefaly device (Cefaly Technology, Grâce-Hollogne, Belgium) delivers transcutaneous electrical stimulation to both supraorbital nerves and is FDA approved in the United States as well.
- Transcranial direct current stimulation: Transcranial direct current stimulation can modulate cortical activity via nodal (activating) or cathodal (inhibition) stimulation that is delivered using a noninvasive portable device.
- Transcranial magnetic stimulation: Transcranial magnetic stimulation (TMS) is a noninvasive technique that uses fluctuating magnetic fields to induce a current in targeted areas of the cerebral cortex. Spring TMS (eNeura Inc., Sunnyvale, CA) is a portable single-pulse device that is approved in the United States for the acute treatment of migraine with aura, but in Europe it is approved for both abortive and preventive treatment of migraine.
- Noninvasive vagal stimulation: The gammaCore device (electroCore LLC, Basking Ridge, NJ) is a handheld device that provides transcutaneous stimulation of the cervical branch of the vagus nerve.

2.8.3 New Medication on the Horizon

The most recent drug(s) currently under development is humanized monoclonal antibodies targeting CGRP. The development of these monoclonal antibodies is directed at both CGRP and its receptors.[39] This class of medication seems to be the most promising of drugs currently under development in terms of effectiveness for migraine patients. However, the long-term

Table 2.1 Fixed-site, fixed-dose method of onabotulinum toxin A injection for chronic migraine

Muscle of head/neck	Dose and number of injection per muscle
Frontalis	20 units divided in 4 sites
Corrugator supercilii	10 units divided in 2 sites
Procerus	5 units divided in 1 site
Temporalis	40 units divided in 8 sites
Occipitalis	30 units divided in 6 sites
Cervical paraspinal group	20 units divided in 4 sites
Trapezius	30 units divided in 6 sites
Total dose	155 units divided in 31 injection sites

safety of these medications can be a limiting factor after these classes of drugs are released to market.

2.8.4 Surgical Treatment

As evidenced, treatment options for migraine, especially in terms of intractable and CM headache is limited. Trigger point deactivation surgery is one of the most promising and effective methods which has minimal adverse effects. Introduced by Guyuron,[40] this method has been in use for more than a decade and is discussed extensively in this book.

References

[1] Steiner TJ, Gretchen L, Birbeck GL, Jensen RH, Katsarava Z, Stovner LJ, Martelletti P. Headache disorders are third cause of disability worldwide. J Headache Pain 2015;16:58

[2] Gibbs TS, Fleischer AB Jr, Feldman SR, Sam MC, O'Donovan CA. Health care utilization in patients with migraine: demographics and patterns of care in the ambulatory setting. Headache 2003;43(4):330–335

[3] GBD 2016 Disease and Injury Incidence and Prevalence Collaborators. Global, regional, and national incidence, prevalence, and years lived with disability for 328 diseases and injuries for 195 countries, 1990–2016: a systematic analysis for the Global Burden of Disease Study 2016. Lancet 2017; 390(10100):1211–1259

[4] Steiner TJ, Stovner LJ, Birbeck GL. Migraine: the seventh disabler. Cephalalgia 2013;33(5):289–290

[5] Lipton RB, Bigal ME, Diamond M, Freitag F, Reed ML, Stewart WF; AMPP Advisory Group. Migraine prevalence, disease burden, and the need for preventive therapy. Neurology 2007;68(5):343–349

[6] Lipton RB, Stewart WF, Scher AI. Epidemiology and economic impact of migraine. Curr Med Res Opin 2001;17(Suppl 1):s4–s12

[7] Miller S, Matharu MS. Migraine is underdiagnosed and undertreated. Practitioner 2014;258(1774): 19–24, 2–3

[8] Minen MT, Loder E, Tishler L, Silbersweig D. Migraine diagnosis and treatment: a knowledge and needs assessment among primary care providers. Cephalalgia 2016;36(4):358–370

[9] Miller VA. Misunderstood and misdiagnosed: the agony of migraine headache. Adv Nurse Pract 2005;13(10):55–56, 58–60, 62

[10] Hawkins K, Wang S, Rupnow MF. Indirect cost burden of migraine in the United States. J Occup Environ Med 2007;49(4):368–374

[11] Hawkins K, Wang S, Rupnow M. Direct cost burden among insured US employees with migraine. Headache 2008;48(4):553–563

[12] Uddman R, Edvinsson L, Ekman R, Kingman T, McCulloch J. Innervation of the feline cerebral vasculature by nerve fibers containing calcitonin gene-related peptide: trigeminal origin and co-existence with substance P. Neurosci Lett 1985;62(1):131–136

[13] Liu Y, Broman J, Edvinsson L. Central projections of sensory innervation of the rat superior sagittal sinus. Neuroscience 2004;129(2):431–437

[14] Durham PL. Diverse physiological roles of calcitonin gene-related peptide in migraine pathology: modulation of neuronal-glial-immune cells to promote peripheral and central sensitization. Curr Pain Headache Rep 2016;20(8):48

[15] Strassman AM, Raymond SA, Burstein R. Sensitization of meningeal sensory neurons and the origin of headaches. Nature 1996;384(6609):560–564

[16] Kelman L. The postdrome of the acute migraine attack. Cephalalgia 2006;26(2):214–220

[17] Kelman L, Tanis D. The relationship between migraine pain and other associated symptoms. Cephalalgia 2006;26(5):548–553

[18] Schoonman GG, Evers DJ, Terwindt GM, van Dijk JG, Ferrari MD. The prevalence of premonitory symptoms in migraine: a questionnaire study in 461 patients. Cephalalgia 2006;26(10):1209–1213

[19] Headache Classification Committee of the International Headache Society (IHS). The International Classification of Headache Disorders. 3rd edition (beta version). Cephalalgia 2013;33(9):629–808

[20] Natoli JL, Manack A, Dean B, et al. Global prevalence of chronic migraine: a systematic review. Cephalalgia 2010;30(5):599–609

[21] Bigal ME, Serrano D, Reed M, Lipton RB. Chronic migraine in the population: burden, diagnosis, and satisfaction with treatment. Neurology 2008;71(8): 559–566

[22] Dodick DW. Clinical practice. Chronic daily headache. N Engl J Med 2006;354(2):158–165

[23] Vos T, Flaxman AD, Naghavi M, et al. Years lived with disability (YLDs) for 1160 sequelae of 289 diseases and injuries 1990-2010: a systematic analysis for the Global Burden of Disease Study 2010. Lancet 2012;380(9859):2163–2196

[24] Depomed, Inc. CAMBIA: Acute Migraine Treatment. Newark, CA: Depomed, Inc.; 2016

[25] Ferrari MD, Roon KI, Lipton RB, Goadsby PJ. Oral triptans (serotonin 5-HT(1B/1D) agonists) in acute migraine treatment: a meta-analysis of 53 trials. Lancet 2001;358(9294):1668–1675

[26] Avanir Pharmaceuticals Inc. ONZETRA® Xsail® (sumatriptan nasal powder): US prescribing information.2016. Available at:https://www.onzetra.com. Accessed September 8, 2016/eref

[27] Feeney R. Medication overuse headache due to butalbital, acetaminophen, and caffeine tablets. J Pain Palliat Care Pharmacother 2016;30(2):148–149

[28] Tfelt-Hansen PC, Diener HC. Why should American headache and migraine patients still be treated with butalbital-containing medicine? Headache 2012;52(4):672–674

[29] Romero CE, Baron JD, Knox AP, Hinchey JA, Ropper AH. Barbiturate withdrawal following Internet purchase of Fioricet. Arch Neurol 2004;61(7): 1111–1112

[30] Tepper SJ, Spears RC. Acute treatment of migraine. Neurol Clin 2009;27(2):417–427

[31] Lipton RB, Silberstein SD. Why study the comorbidity of migraine? Neurology 1994;44(10, Suppl 7):S4–S5

[32] Silberstein SD, Winner PK, Chmiel JJ. Migraine preventive medication reduces resource utilization. Headache 2003;43(3):171–178

[33] Lipton RB, Diamond M, Freitag F, et al. Migraine prevention patterns in a community sample: results from American migraine prevalence and prevention (AMPP)study. Headache 2005;45:792–793

[34] Ansari H, Ziad S. Drug-drug interactions in headache medicine. Headache 2016;56(7):1241–1248

[35] Aurora SK, Dodick DW, Turkel CC, et al; PREEMPT 1 Chronic Migraine Study Group. Onabotulinum toxin A for treatment of chronic migraine: results from the double-blind, randomized, placebo-controlled phase of the PREEMPT 1 trial. Cephalalgia 2010;30(7): 793–803

[36] Diener HC, Dodick DW, Aurora SK, et al; PREEMPT 2 Chronic Migraine Study Group. OnabotulinumtoxinA for treatment of chronic migraine: results from the double-blind, randomized, placebo-controlled phase of the PREEMPT 2 trial. Cephalalgia 2010;30(7): 804–814

[37] Ashkenazi A, Levin M, Dodick DW. Peripheral procedures: nerve blocks, peripheral neurostimulation and botulinum neurotoxin injections. In: Silberstein SD, Lipton RB, Dodick DW, eds. Wolff's Headache and Other Head Pain. New York, NY: Oxford University Press;2007:767–792

[38] Ashkenazi A, Matro R, Shaw JW, Abbas MA, Silberstein SD. Greater occipital nerve block using local anaesthetics alone or with triamcinolone for transformed migraine: a randomised comparative study. J Neurol Neurosurg Psychiatry 2008;79(4): 415–417

[39] Schuster NM, Rapoport AM. New strategies for the treatment and prevention of primary headache disorders. Nat Rev Neurol 2016;12(11):635–650

[40] Guyuron B. Surgical management of migraine headaches.In: Achauer BM, Eriksson E, Guyuron B, Coleman JJ III, Russell RC, Vander Kolk CA, eds.Plastic Surgery: Indications, Operations, and Outcomes. St. Louis, Mo: Mosby;2000:281–291

3   Surgical Anatomy of the Frontal and Occipital Trigger Sites

Jeffrey E. Janis and Ibrahim Khansa

Salient Points

- The frontal trigger site includes the supraorbital and supratrochlear nerves (STN). Both nerves are derived from the frontal nerve, which is the largest branch of the ophthalmic division of the trigeminal nerve (V1).

- Eighty-three percent of individuals have a notch, 27% have a foramen, and 10% have both.

- The supraorbital notch contains a fascial band 86% of the time.

- When a supraorbital foramen is present, it is located on average 31 mm lateral to the midline,[1] although this location is inconsistent and can be asymmetric even between the two sides of a single individual.

- After passing through the supraorbital notch or foramen, the SON divides into a deep branch and a superficial branch. The deep branch is located approximately 0.56 mm lateral to a vertical line through the medial limbus.

- The deep branch of the supraorbital nerve (SON) is susceptible to compression inferolaterally.

- As they travel cranially, one or both branches of the SON course directly through the corrugator supercilii muscle (CSM) in 78% of individuals.

- Supraorbital artery travels medial to the SON.

- The STN usually divides into two branches in the retro-orbicularis fat.

- Similar to the SON, one or both branches of the STN may travel through the CSM, which comprises a potential compression or trigger point of the supratrochlear.

- In 84% of individuals, both branches of the STN enter the CSM 18.8 mm lateral to the midline, and exit it 19.6 mm lateral to the midline and 15 mm cranial to the superior orbital rim.[2]

- The occipital trigger site comprises three sets of nerves, constituting three distinct trigger sites, one medially along the posterior midline (the third occipital), one about 1.5 cm lateral to the midline (greater occipital), and one laterally close to the hairline (the lesser occipital).

- The greater occipital artery can be compressed or irritated at six sites.

- The greater occipital nerve (GON) travels around the lower border of the obliquus capitis inferior muscle, where fascial bands between this muscle and the nerve constitute the first potential compression point of the GON.

- The entrance of the GON into the deep aspect (undersurface) of the semispinalis capitis muscle constitutes the second potential compression point, located 17.5 mm lateral and 59.7 mm caudal to the occipital protuberance.

- The emergence of the GON from the superficial aspect of the semispinalis capitis muscle constitutes the third potential compression point, located 15.5 mm lateral and 34.5 mm caudal to the external occipital protuberance (EOP).

- The GON then continues cranially deep to the trapezius muscle, before entering the deep surface, the fourth potential compression point.[3]

- The GON then emerges from the tendinous insertion of the trapezius into the nuchal line, at a point 37.1 mm lateral and 4.4 mm caudal to the EOP, and this constitutes the fifth potential compression point.[3]

- The GON intersects with the occipital artery in 54 to 64% of individuals,[4,5] and this intersection constitutes the sixth potential compression point.

- The lesser occipital nerve emerges around the posterior border of the sternocleidomastoid muscle in 86.7% of individuals,[6] or through the muscle in the remaining 13.3% of individuals, and this constitutes the first potential compression point.

- The lesser occipital compression point is located 61.3 to 68.9 mm lateral to the midline, and 53.2 mm below the level of the external auditory canals.

- The lesser occipital nerve intersects with the occipital artery in 55% of individuals,[7] and this constitutes the second potential compression point, located 51 mm lateral to the midline and 20 mm caudal to the level of the external auditory canal.

3.1 Introduction

The anatomy of the frontal and occipital trigger sites has been studied extensively as it pertains to possible contributions to migraine headaches. Each of these trigger sites includes several potential trigger points that highlight the wide variety of structures that may interact with sensory nerves to produce headache symptoms, including muscle, bone, fascia, and vessel. In this chapter, the anatomy of the supraorbital, supratrochlear, greater occipital, third occipital, and lesser occipital nerves (LON) is detailed, including all known compression and irritation points.

3.2 Frontal Trigger Site

The frontal trigger site includes the supraorbital nerve (SON) and supratrochlear nerve (STN). Both nerves are derived from the frontal nerve, which is the largest branch of the ophthalmic division of the trigeminal nerve (V1). It also includes muscle, particularly the corrugator supercilii, the procerus, and depressor supercilii, as well as bone, fascia, and vessel.

3.2.1 Supraorbital Nerve

The SON may exit the orbit through a notch in the supraorbital rim or through a foramen just cranial to the rim, and this notch or foramen constitutes the first potential compression point of the SON. Fallucco et al found that individuals are most likely to have a supraorbital notch than a foramen (83% of individuals have a notch, 27% have a foramen, and 10% have both).[2] In a separate anatomical study, Webster et al found bilateral supraorbital notches in 50% of individuals, bilateral supraorbital foramina in 25% of individuals, and a notch on one side with a foramen on the contralateral side in 25% of individuals.[8] When a supraorbital notch is present, it is located on average 25 mm lateral to the midline.[9] The notch

contains a fascial band 86% of the time. Fallucco et al divided those fascial bands into three types[2]: type I bands (51.2%) consist of a single fascial band at the caudal edge of the notch. Type II bands (30.2%) consist of bony spicules and a fascial band at the caudal edge of the notch. Type III bands (18.6%) consist of a septum within the notch that creates multiple passageways for the neurovascular bundle (▶Fig. 3.1). When a supraorbital foramen is present, it is located on average 31 mm lateral to the midline,[1] although this location is inconsistent and can be asymmetric even between the two sides of a single individual. The location of the foramen also varies by gender (more lateral in males)[10] and by race (more lateral in Blacks).[11]

After passing through the supraorbital notch or foramen, the SON divides into a deep branch and a superficial branch. The deep branch is located approximately 0.56 mm lateral to a vertical line through the medial limbus.[12] Both branches may interact with the corrugator supercilii muscle (CSM) at multiple points, and precise knowledge of the location and topography of the CSM is essential to achieve adequate chemodenervation or surgical resection of this muscle. In the transverse plane, the CSM extends from approximately 3 mm lateral to the vertical midline to a distance approximately 85% of the distance to the lateral orbital rim. The apex of the muscle is located approximately 33 mm above the horizontal plane drawn between the nasion and lateral orbital rim at the level of the lateral limbus (▶Fig. 3.2).[13]

Along its inferior free border, the CSM is surrounded by a galeal fat pad,[14] and nerve compression there is unlikely due to this padding. However, inferolaterally, the CSM interdigitates with the orbicularis oculi muscle, and the deep branch of the SON is susceptible to compression there due to repetitive muscle contraction.[13] An additional potential compression point of the deep branch of the SON occurs when it changes direction from its firmly adherent location on the periosteum to a more superficial plane, leading to a potential kink in the nerve.[13]

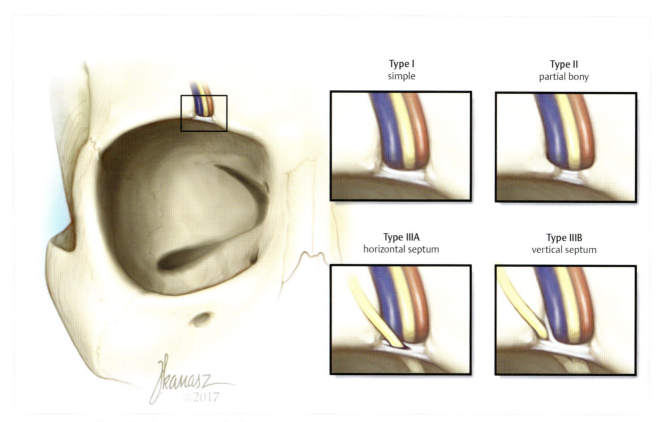

Fig. 3.1 Types of fascial bands at the supraorbital notch.

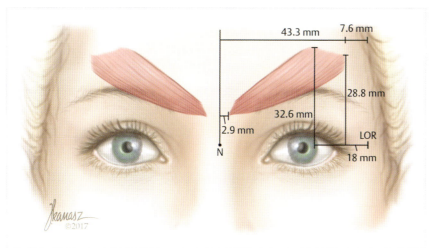

Fig. 3.2 Topography of the corrugator supercilii muscle.

As they travel cranially, one or both branches of the SON course directly through the CSM in 78% of individuals.[13,15] The branching pattern of the SON in relation to the CSM has been studied by Janis et al, who identified four patterns[15]: a type I pattern (40%), where branches off the deep branch of the SON (SON-D) travels through the CSM, a type II pattern (34%), where branches off both the superficial (SON-S) and deep branches of the SON travel through the CSM, a type III pattern (4%), where branches off the SON-S travel through the CSM, and a type IV pattern (22%) where there are no branches from either the SON-D or SON-S that travel through the CSM (▶ Fig. 3.3).

More cranially, the horizontal fibers of the CSM interdigitate with the vertical fibers of the frontalis muscle, and those opposing muscle forces may apply torque to one or both branches of the SON, leading to compression.[15]

After passing through or deep to the CSM, the deep branch of the SON travels cranially in the layer between the galea aponeurotica and the periosteum to provide sensory innervation to the frontoparietal scalp. The superficial branch of the SON divides into multiple smaller branches that pierce the frontalis muscle before reaching the subcutaneous tissue and skin of the lateral forehead.[15,16] The supraorbital artery travels with the SON and often it is located medial to it.

3.2.2 Supratrochlear Nerve

The STN exits the orbit via either a notch or a foramen, located 16 to 23 mm lateral to the midline, which is more medial that the exit point of the SON.[17] The foramen is exceedingly rare. Unlike SON, this notch or foramen rarely constitutes a potential compression point of the STN.

The STN usually divides into two branches in the retro-orbicularis fat. Similar to the SON, one or both branches of the STN may travel through the CSM, which comprises the second potential compression point of the STN. In 84% of individuals, both branches of the STN enter the CSM 18.8 mm lateral to the midline, and exit it 19.6 mm lateral to the midline and 15 mm cranial to the superior orbital rim.[18] In 4% of individuals, one branch of the STN travels through the CSM, while the other stays deep to the plane of the muscle, and in 12% of individuals, both branches of the STN remain deep to the CSM at all times with neither branch traveling through it (▶ Fig. 3.4).

Similar to the SON, the branches of the STN may also be compressed by the interdigitations between the horizontal CSM fibers and the vertical frontalis muscle fibers.[15] After traveling through or deep to the CSM, the branches of the STN pierce the frontalis muscle to provide sensory innervation to the subcutaneous tissue and skin of the midline forehead. The supratrochlear accompanies the STN.

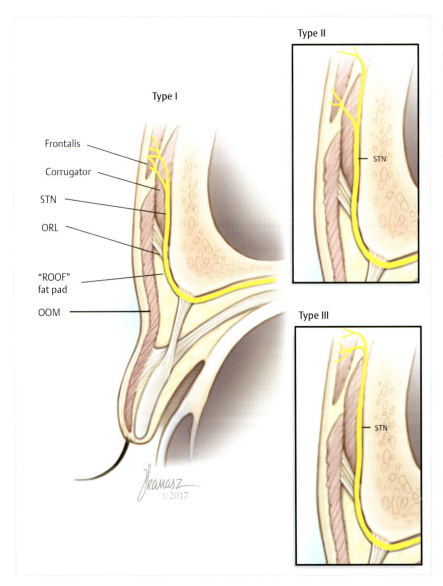

Fig. 3.3 Branching patterns of the supraorbital nerve in relation to the corrugator supercilii muscle. SON-S, superficial division of the supraorbital nerve; SON-S$_{CSM}$, branch of the superficial division of the supraorbital nerve traveling through the corrugator supercilii muscle; SON-D, deep division of the supraorbital nerve; SON-D$_{CSM}$, branch of the deep division of the supraorbital nerve traveling through the corrugator supercilii muscle.

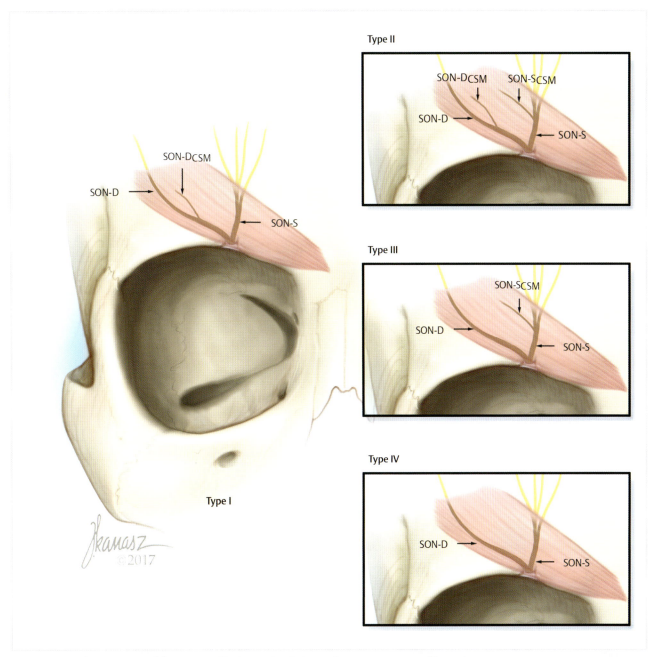

Fig. 3.4 Branching patterns of the supratrochlear nerve in relation to the corrugator supercilii muscle.

3.3 Occipital Trigger Site

The occipital trigger site comprises three sets of nerves, constituting three distinct trigger sites, one medially along the posterior midline (the third occipital), one about 1.5 cm lateral to the midline (the greater occipital), and one laterally close to the hairline (the third occipital). The greater occipital nerve (GON) derives from the dorsal ramus of the C2 spinal nerve,[19] while the third occipital nerve derives from the dorsal ramus of the C3 spinal nerve.[6] The LON derives from the ventral rami of the C2 and C3 spinal nerves.[6]

3.3.1 Greater Occipital Nerve

The GON has been extensively studied, and was the first peripheral nerve focused on as it pertains to its contributions to migraine headaches in 2004.[20] Ultimately, driven by clinical failures to adequately decompress this nerve, further investigation was performed that recognized that there were six different points of potential GON compression, rather than just one.[3]

After emerging from the dorsal ramus of the C2 spinal nerve, the GON travels in a caudal, posterior, and lateral direction, around the lower border of the obliquus capitis inferior muscle, where fascial bands between this muscle and the nerve constitute the first potential compression point of the GON. This compression point is located 20.1 mm lateral and 77.4 mm caudal to the external occipital protuberance (EOP; ▶ Fig. 3.5).[3]

The nerve then continues in a cranial direction, superficial to the obliquus capitis inferior muscle and deep to the semispinalis capitis muscle. It pierces the semispinalis capitis muscle and crosses it from deep to superficial in 90% of individuals.[21] The entrance of the GON into the deep aspect (undersurface) of the semispinalis capitis muscle constitutes the second potential compression point, located 17.5 mm lateral and 59.7 mm caudal to the EOP.

The emergence of the GON from the superficial aspect of the semispinalis capitis muscle constitutes the third potential compression point, located

15.5 mm lateral and 34.5 mm caudal to the EOP. Other authors have confirmed the approximate location of this important compression point as 1.5 cm lateral and 3 cm caudal to the EOP.[21,22]

The GON then continues cranially deep to the trapezius muscle, before entering the deep surface of the muscle 24 mm lateral and 21 mm caudal to the EOP. This entrance into the trapezius, known as the trapezial tunnel, constitutes the fourth potential compression point.[3]

The GON then emerges from the tendinous insertion of the trapezius into the nuchal line, at a point 37.1 mm lateral and 4.4 mm caudal to the EOP, and this constitutes the fifth potential compression point.[3]

The GON intersects with the occipital artery in 54 to 64% of individuals,[4,5] and this intersection constitutes the sixth potential compression point. This

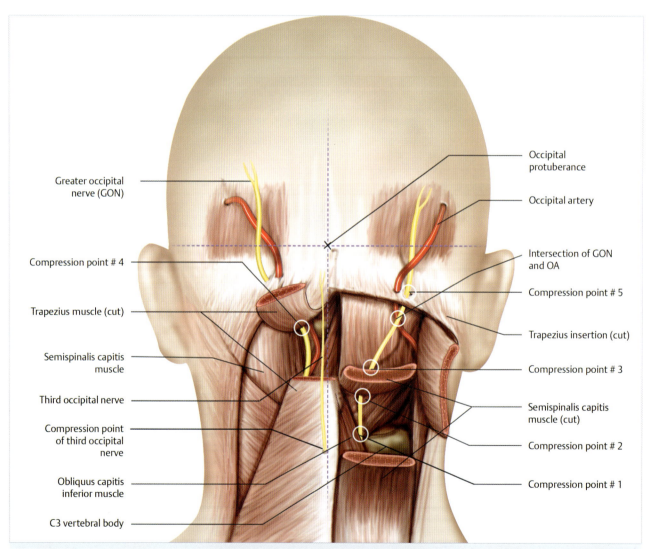

Fig. 3.5 Course and compression points of the greater occipital, third occipital, and lesser occipital nerves. (Reproduced with permission from Khansa I, Barker JC, Janis JE. Sensory nerves of the head and neck. In: Watanabe K, Shoja MM, Loukas M, Tubbs RS, eds. Anatomical Basis of Plastic Surgery of the Head and Neck. New York, NY: Thieme; 2016:86–100.)

compression point is quite variable and may even occur proximal to the fifth compression point. The interaction between the GON and the occipital artery takes the form of a simple intersection in 29.6% of cases, located 30.3 mm lateral and 10.7 mm caudal to the EOP. The interaction may also take the form of a helical intertwining over a distance of 37.6 mm in the remaining 70.4% of individuals, spanning from 25.3 to 42.09 mm lateral and 1.0 to 24.9 mm caudal to the EOP.[3]

In a large anatomic study of live patients and cadavers, Ducic et al corroborated the location of the GON exit from the semispinalis muscle.[22] They also highlighted some variations in the anatomy of the GON. In 6.1% of individuals, semispinalis muscle fibers actually split the nerve into two fibers, which then reconnect superficial to the muscle. In 43.9% of individuals, the course of the GON is asymmetric between the two sides.

After emerging from the trapezius, the GON continues traveling cranially to provide sensory innervation to the medial posterior scalp.

3.3.2 Lesser Occipital Nerve

The LON emerges around the posterior border of the sternocleidomastoid (SCM) muscle in 86.7% of individuals,[6] or through the muscle in the remaining 13.3% of individuals, and this constitutes the first potential compression point of the LON (▶ Fig. 3.5). This compression point is located 61.3 to 68.9 mm lateral to the midline and 53.2 mm below the level of the external auditory canals.

The LON then travels superolaterally along the posterior border of the SCM. It intersects with the occipital artery in 55% of individuals,[7] and this constitutes the second potential compression point, located 51 mm lateral to the midline and 20 mm caudal to the level of the external auditory canal. Eighty-two percent of those cases consist of a simple intersection. The remaining 18% consist of a helical intertwining between the LON and the occipital artery.[6]

Twenty percent of individuals have a third compression point, consisting of a fascial band located 47 mm lateral to the midline and 13.1 mm inferior to the level of the external auditory canal.[7] The nerve branches into a medial component that provides sensory innervation to the superior ear and postauricular skin, and a lateral component that provides sensory innervation to the lateral neck.

3.3.3 Third Occipital Nerve

The TON is located inferior to the GON and always emerges through the semispinalis capitis muscle.

This first potential compression point is located 13 mm lateral to the midline and 60 mm caudal to the external auditory canals, or roughly 3 cm inferior to the GON (▶ Fig. 3.5).[6] The location of this compression point is quite variable.[23]

After piercing the semispinalis capitis muscle, the TON continues cranially to provide sensory innervation to the posterior medial scalp and neck. The TON has several interconnections with the GON and the contralateral TON. It is smaller than the GON, travels in a more deep to superficial trajectory, and does not have as many points of possible compression.

3.4 Conclusion

Numerous anatomical studies have helped elucidate the detailed anatomy of the nerves involved in the frontal and occipital trigger points. Knowledge of the precise course and potential compression points of these nerves is essential to full and effective decompression.

References

[1] Beer GM, Putz R, Mager K, Schumacher M, Keil W. Variations of the frontal exit of the supraorbital nerve: an anatomic study. Plast Reconstr Surg 1998;102(2):334–341

[2] Fallucco M, Janis JE, Hagan RR. The anatomical morphology of the supraorbital notch: clinical relevance to the surgical treatment of migraine headaches. Plast Reconstr Surg 2012;130(6):1227–1233

[3] Janis JE, Hatef DA, Ducic I, et al. The anatomy of the greater occipital nerve: part II. Compression point topography. Plast Reconstr Surg 2010;126(5): 1563–1572

[4] Janis JE, Hatef DA, Reece EM, McCluskey PD, Schaub TA, Guyuron B. Neurovascular compression of the greater occipital nerve: implications for migraine headaches. Plast Reconstr Surg 2010;126(6): 1996–2001

[5] Junewicz A, Katira K, Guyuron B. Intraoperative anatomical variations during greater occipital nerve decompression. J Plast Reconstr Aesthet Surg 2013;66(10):1340–1345

[6] Dash KS, Janis JE, Guyuron B. The lesser and third occipital nerves and migraine headaches. Plast Reconstr Surg 2005;115(6):1752–1758, discussion 1759–1760

[7] Lee M, Brown M, Chepla K, et al. An anatomical study of the lesser occipital nerve and its potential compression points: implications for surgical treatment of migraine headaches. Plast Reconstr Surg 2013;132(6):1551–1556

[8] Webster RC, Gaunt JM, Hamdan US, Fuleihan NS, Giandello PR, Smith RC. Supraorbital and supratrochlear notches and foramina: anatomical

variations and surgical relevance. Laryngoscope 1986;96(3):311–315

[9] Saylam C, Ozer MA, Ozek C, Gurler T. Anatomical variations of the frontal and supraorbital transcranial passages. J Craniofac Surg 2003;14(1):10–12

[10] Agthong S, Huanmanop T, Chentanez V. Anatomical variations of the supraorbital, infraorbital, and mental foramina related to gender and side. J Oral Maxillofac Surg 2005;63(6):800–804

[11] Cutright B, Quillopa N, Schubert W. An anthropometric analysis of the key foramina for maxillofacial surgery. J Oral Maxillofac Surg 2003;61(3):354–357

[12] Cuzalina AL, Holmes JD. A simple and reliable landmark for identification of the supraorbital nerve in surgery of the forehead: an in vivo anatomical study. J Oral Maxillofac Surg 2005;63(1):25–27

[13] Janis JE, Ghavami A, Lemmon JA, Leedy JE, Guyuron B. Anatomy of the corrugator supercilii muscle: part I. Corrugator topography. Plast Reconstr Surg 2007;120(6):1647–1653

[14] Knize DM. Muscles that act on glabellar skin: a closer look. Plast Reconstr Surg 2000;105(1):350–361

[15] Janis JE, Ghavami A, Lemmon JA, Leedy JE, Guyuron B. The anatomy of the corrugator supercilii muscle: part II. Supraorbital nerve branching patterns. Plast Reconstr Surg 2008;121(1):233–240

[16] Knize DM. Transpalpebral approach to the corrugator supercilii and procerus muscles. Plast Reconstr Surg 1995;95(1):52–60, discussion 61–62

[17] Miller TA, Rudkin G, Honig M, Elahi M, Adams J. Lateral subcutaneous brow lift and interbrow muscle resection: clinical experience and anatomic studies. Plast Reconstr Surg 2000;105(3):1120–1127, discussion 1128

[18] Janis JE, Hatef DA, Hagan R, et al. Anatomy of the supratrochlear nerve: implications for the surgical treatment of migraine headaches. Plast Reconstr Surg 2013;131(4):743–750

[19] Ducic I, Hartmann EC, Larson EE. Indications and outcomes for surgical treatment of patients with chronic migraine headaches caused by occipital neuralgia. Plast Reconstr Surg 2009;123(5):1453–1461

[20] Mosser SW, Guyuron B, Janis JE, Rohrich RJ. The anatomy of the greater occipital nerve: implications for the etiology of migraine headaches. Plast Reconstr Surg 2004;113(2):693–697, discussion 698–700

[21] Bovim G, Bonamico L, Fredriksen TA, Lindboe CF, Stolt-Nielsen A, Sjaastad O. Topographic variations in the peripheral course of the greater occipital nerve. Autopsy study with clinical correlations. Spine 1991;16(4):475–478

[22] Ducic I, Moriarty M, Al-Attar A. Anatomical variations of the occipital nerves: implications for the treatment of chronic headaches. Plast Reconstr Surg 2009;123(3):859–863, discussion 864

[23] Tubbs RS, Mortazavi MM, Loukas M, et al. Anatomical study of the third occipital nerve and its potential role in occipital headache/neck pain following midline dissections of the craniocervical junction. J Neurosurg Spine 2011;15(1):71–75

4 Surgical Anatomy of the Temporal Migraine Headaches

Ali Totonchi

Salient Points

- The trigeminal ganglion is the main source of sensory supply for the majority of the face, including the temporal area.
- The maxillary branch of the trigeminal nerve leaves the cranium through the foramen rotundum and enters the pterygopalatine fossa.
- After providing branches to the pterygopalatine ganglion, it divides into the infraorbital and the zygomatic nerves.
- The zygomatic nerve leans toward the lateral orbital wall and divides into the zygomaticotemporal and the zygomaticofacial branches.
- The temporal and malar areas are supplied by the zygomaticotemporal and the auriculotemporal nerve branches.
- The zygomatic nerve is divided into the zygomaticotemporal and the zygomaticofacial nerves inside the orbit; each of these nerves passes through the malar bone.
- The zygomaticotemporal branch of the trigeminal nerve (ZTBTN) enters the temporal fossa deep to the temporalis muscle.
- After entering the temporal fossa, the ZTBTN travels toward the surface of the muscle and pierces the deep temporal fascia.
- The nerve exits the deep temporal fascia 16 to 17 mm lateral and 6.5 mm cephalic to the later canthus.
- The ZTBTN does not travel within the muscle in 50% of the study specimens.
- The auriculotemporal nerve branches from the main mandibular trunk after it exits the foramen ovale.
- After exiting the foramen, the nerve divides into two roots that go around the middle meningeal artery and then unite under the lateral pterygoid muscles on the surface of the tensor veli palatini.
- The nerve then passes between sphenomandibular ligament and the neck of the mandible and then runs laterally behind the temporomandibular joint toward the upper portion of the parotid gland.
- The nerve travels superficially at the level of the temporoparietal fascia caudally and the subcutaneous tissue cephalically.
- In the temporal region, the nerve is divided into the anterior and posterior branches and is accompanied by the superficial temporal artery and vein.
- There is a watershed effect between the anterior branch of the trigeminal nerve and the posterior branch of the ZTBTN.

4.1 Introduction

The temporal area is one of the most common trigger sites for migraine headaches. Since the introduction of migraine surgery in the early 2000s, our understanding of the anatomy of the nervous system in this area and its contribution to migraine headache and subsequently the surgical techniques for its treatment has evolved. There are a few small sensory nerves in the temple area that can trigger migraine headaches. A clear understanding of soft-tissue anatomy and facial and trigeminal nerve branches, along with safe surgical access to this area, plays an integral role in successful and safe surgery.

4.2 Central Nervous System Anatomy

The trigeminal ganglion is the main source of sensory supply for the majority of the face, including the temporal area; it spans from the superior part of pons to the medulla (▶ Fig. 4.1). This nucleus has a small motor portion, which supplies the muscles of mastication, mylohyoid, anterior belly of digastric muscle, tensor veli palatini, and tensor tympani.

The sensory part of the nuclei, which is the topic of this chapter, constitutes the majority of the nucleus.

The nerve leaves the brain in separate sensory and motor bundles with the sensory bundle being significantly larger than the motor bundle. Next, the sensory branch enters the trigeminal ganglion and the ganglion gives three branches:

• **The ophthalmic nerve (V1)** leaves the cranium through the superior orbital fissure and continues to the frontal nerve. It also branches to the nasociliary ganglion and lacrimal gland.
The frontal branch divides itself into the supraorbital and supratrochlear nerves, which travel under the orbital roof to the orbital rim. These nerves will be discussed in a separate chapter.

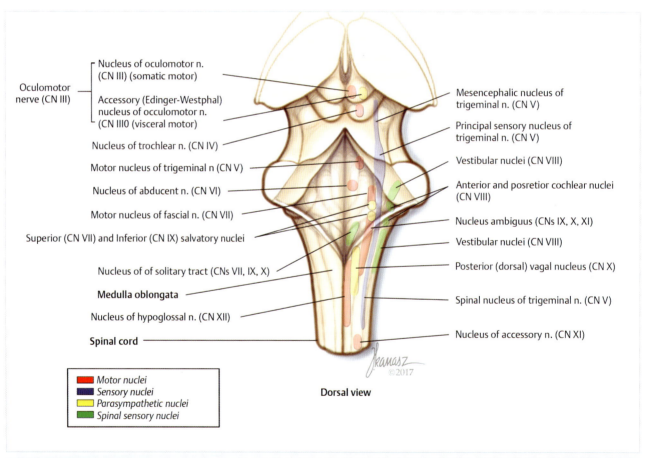

Fig. 4.1 Trigeminal nucleus.

- **The maxillary nerve (V2)** leaves the cranium through the foramen rotundum and enters the pterygopalatine fossa. After providing branches to the pterygopalatine ganglion, it divides into the infraorbital and zygomatic nerves. The zygomatic nerve leans toward the lateral orbital wall and divides into the zygomaticotemporal and zygomaticofacial branches.
- **The mandibular nerve (V3)** leaves the cranium through the foramen ovale, medial to the temporomandibular joint, and divides into the lingual, buccal, and inferior alveolar auriculotemporal nerves.

Motor branches also leave the cranium through the foramen ovale and supply muscles of mastication.

4.3 Temporal Area Soft-Tissue Anatomy

The temporalis muscle lies on the temporal fossa, starting from the coronoid process of the mandible traveling cephalically and passing under the zygomatic arch and attaching to the bone like a fan over the inferior temporal line. This muscle is covered by a complex structure composed of fascia, fat pads, and the temporal branch of the facial nerves (▶ Fig 4.2).

The deepest layer is the deep temporal fascia, which starts from the inferior temporal line and travels caudally; in the halfway between the temporal line and zygomatic arch, it divides into superficial and deep layers of the deep temporal fascia. These two layers of the deep temporal fascia contain the deep temporal fat pad. Superficial to the superficial layer of the deep temporal fascia is a loose areolar tissue. This tissue is directly under the superficial layer of the temporal fascia, which is the continuation of the superficial musculoaponeurotic system (SMAS) layer. The temporal branch of the facial nerve passes deep to the SMAS at the level of the zygomatic arch.

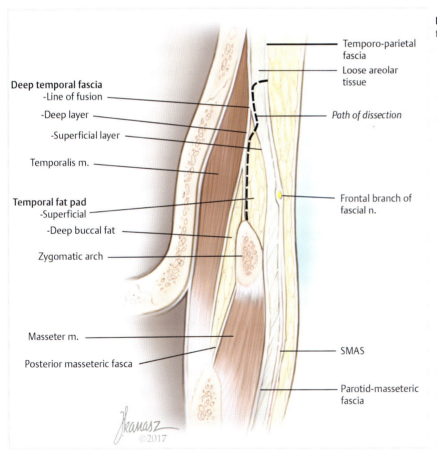

Fig. 4.2 Soft-tissue anatomy of the temporal area.

4.4 Temporal Area Sensory Nervous Supply

The temporal and malar areas are supplied by zygomatic and auriculotemporal nerve branches. The zygomatic nerve is divided into zygomaticotemporal and zygomaticofacial nerves inside orbit. Each of these nerves passes through the malar bone; the zygomaticotemporal branch of the trigeminal nerve (ZTBTN) enters the temporal fossa deep to the temporalis muscle, while the zygomaticofacial branch of the trigeminal nerve (ZFBTN) passes through the malar bone and comes to the surface at the anterolateral part of the cheekbones. Unlike ZFBTN, which rarely acts as a trigger site, ZFBTN is one of the most common trigger sites in the migraine headache (▶Fig 4.3).

After ZTBTN enters the temporal fossa, it travels toward the surface of the muscle and pierces the deep temporal fascia. Our studies have demonstrated that this nerve exits the fascia 16 to 17 mm (average of 16.8 mm on the right side and 17.1 mm on the left side) lateral and 6.5 mm cephalic (average of 6.6 cm on left side and 6.4 mm on the right side) to the lateral canthus (▶Fig. 4.4, ▶Fig. 4.5).[1] Same study showed three major accessory branches of the nerve, classified as (1) branches adjacent to the main branch, (2) branches lateral to the main branch, and (3) branches cephalic to the main branch. Another study performed by Janis et al showed that in 50% of the specimen ZTBTN remains between the muscle and the temporal bone and does not enter the muscle; in 22%, there is a short straight course in the muscle; and in 28%, the nerve had a long tortuous course inside the muscle.[2]

4.5 Auriculotemporal Nerve

The auriculotemporal nerve branches from the main mandibular trunk after it exits the foramen ovale. After exiting the foramen, the nerve divides into two roots that go around the middle meningeal artery and then unite under the lateral pterygoid muscles on the surface of the tensor veli palatini. The nerve then passes between the sphenomandibular ligament and the neck of the mandible and then runs laterally behind the temporomandibular joint toward upper portion of the parotid gland. The nerve travels superficially at the level of the temporoparietal fascia caudally and the subcutaneous tissue cephalically. In the temporal region, the nerve is divided into anterior and posterior branches, and it is accompanied by the superficial temporal artery and vein. There is a watershed effect between the anterior branch of the trigeminal nerve and the posterior branch of the ZTBTN.

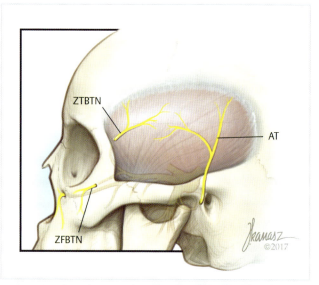

Fig. 4.3 Illustration of the zygomaticotemporal branch of the trigeminal nerve. AT, auriculotemporal; ZTBTN, zygomaticotemporal branch of the trigeminal nerve; ZFTBN, zygomaticofacial branch of the trigeminal nerve.

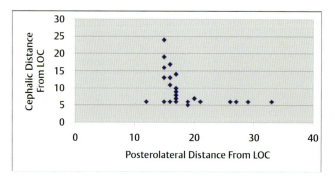

Fig. 4.4 Right-sided measurements of the zygomaticotemporal branches of the trigeminal nerve (ZTBTN) from lateral canthus. (Adapted from Totonchi et al.[1])

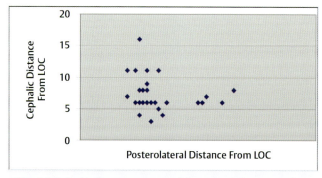

Fig. 4.5 Left-sided measurements of the zygomaticotemporal branches of the trigeminal nerve (ZTBTN) from lateral canthus. (Adapted from Totonchi et al.[1])

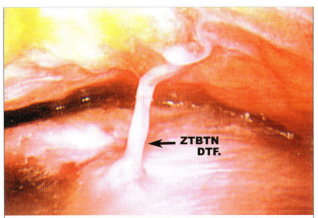

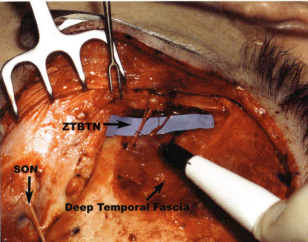

Fig. 4.6 Endoscopic (top) and open (bottom) views of the Zygomaticotemporal branch of trigeminal nerve (ZTBTN) and deep temporal fascia. (Adapted from Totonchi et al.[1])

4.6 Conclusion

Temporal area is supplied by the zygomaticotemporal and auriculotemporal nerves, in general the hair bearing area supplied by the auriculotemporal nerve and the non-hair-bearing area supplied by the ZTBTN (▶ Fig. 4.6). Understanding the anatomy of the nerves, the temporal fascia, and the temporal branch of the facial nerve will help in proper execution of the surgery and protecting the motor branch of the nerve.

References

[1] Totonchi A, Pashmini N, Guyuron B. The zygomatico-temporal branch of the trigeminal nerve: an anatomical study. Plast Reconstr Surg 2005;115(1):273–277

[2] Janis JE, Hatef DA, Thakar H, et al. The zygomaticotemporal branch of the trigeminal nerve: part II. Anatomical variations. Plast Reconstr Surg 2010;126(2):435–442

5 Evidence for Efficacy of Migraine Surgery

Bahman Guyuron

Salient Points

- The first research on current migraine surgery was prompted by two patients who reported their migraine headaches (MHs) ceased after a forehead rejuvenation.

- A retrospective study on 314 patients who had undergone forehead rejuvenation demonstrated improvement or elimination of MH in 31 of 39 patients with MH.

- Twenty-one of the 22 patients in a prospective pilot study demonstrated either complete elimination (11 patients) or significant improvement (10 patients) of MH.

- Anatomical study on 20 fresh cadavers demonstrated passage of the greater occipital nerve through the muscle in all and emergence of the nerve from the muscle at a point about 3 cm caudal to the occipital tuberosity and 1.5 cm lateral to the midline.

- A study on 20 patients concluded that the main zygomaticotemporal branch of the trigeminal nerve emerges from the deep temporal fascia on average 17 mm lateral and 6 mm cephalad to the lateral palpebral commissure.

- In a level II randomized study, 82 of the 89 patients (92%) in the treatment group demonstrated at least 50% reduction in MH frequency, duration, or intensity compared to baseline; 31 (35%) reported elimination and 51 (57%) experienced improvement over a mean follow-up period of 396 days.

- In a level II 5-year follow-up study, 61 of 69 (88%) patients continued to have a positive response to the surgery ($p < 0.0001$). Twenty (29%) reported complete elimination of MH and 41 (59%) noticed a significant decrease in frequency, severity, and duration of MH ($p < 0.0001$).

- In a level I randomized study with sham surgery control, 41 of the 49 (83%) patients benefitted from the real surgery compared to 15 of 26 (56%) patients in the sham surgery group ($p = 0.014$). While 28 (57%) patients in the real surgery group observed complete elimination of MH, only 1 patient in the sham surgery group reported elimination ($p < 0.0001$).

- In a level III study, two independent departments at Case Western Reserve University (Center for Proteomics and Bioinformatics and Department of Neurosciences) compared the nerves of the patients with MH to those without and concluded that the nerves of patients with MH had myelin deficit.

- Through a level III study, it was demonstrated that the factors associated with migraine surgery failure include increased intraoperative bleeding and surgery on fewer trigger sites.

- In a level III study, it was discovered that the factors associated with migraine surgery success include older age of migraine onset, presence of visual symptoms, surgery at site I or II, and deactivation of all four common MH sites.

- A level III study demonstrated that there was no statistically significant difference between the injection of botulinum toxin type A and the use of a constellation of symptoms to identify the migraine trigger sites.

- A level III study demonstrated superior outcomes with supraorbital foraminotomy when indicated.

- A level III cost analysis study demonstrated total median cost reduction in migraine care of $3,949.70 per year postoperatively. The mean surgical cost was $8,378.

31

- Through a level III study, it was discovered that endoscopic nerve decompression was more successful in reducing or eliminating frontal MH than transpalpebral nerve decompression.

- -Another level III study verified that a positive botulinum toxin type A response is a significant predictor of migraine surgery success.

- A level III comparative study between those who were on narcotic analgesics and those who avoided these products demonstrated that the group that consumed narcotics had significantly lower rates of improvement from the surgery in all migraine indices.

- In a level III comparative study of surgery outcome on patients with episodic, chronic, and daily MHs, it was discovered that all cohorts, regardless of their frequency of MHs, achieved significant improvement in frequency, duration, severity, and MH index.

- We demonstrated that Doppler signal in the site of most intense pain can predictably confirm the presence of an artery in the most painful site and lead to precise location of the nerve irritation by a vessel and thus a successful removal of the offending artery.

- A level II prospective randomized study concluded that neurectomy and decompression of the zygomaticotemporal branch of the trigeminal nerve are both appropriate treatments for temporal MH.

- A level V retrospective review of an adolescent population has shown that migraine surgery may offer symptomatic improvement of MH frequency, duration, and severity in patients with identifiable anatomical trigger sites.

- In an anatomical study, the location of emergence of the lesser occipital nerve from the trapezius fascia was determined to be an area centered 65.4 ± 11.6 mm from midline and 53.3 ± 15.6 mm caudal to the line connecting the external auditory canals.

- The third occipital nerve was found 13.2 ± 5.3 mm from the midline and 62.0 ± 20.0 mm caudal to the line between the two external auditory canals.

- In another anatomical study, three patterns of interaction were found between the superficial temporal artery and auriculotemporal branch of the trigeminal: a single site where the artery is crossing over the nerve (62.5%), a helical intertwining relationship (18.8%), and nerve crossing over the artery (18.8%).

5.1 Introduction

While the initial reports from two patients indicating that their migraine headaches (MHs) had disappeared following cosmetic surgery were intriguing, one could not help being skeptical about the connection between cosmetic forehead procedures and migraine symptom disappearance. This onset rules out the possibility that the positive outcomes are related to a placebo effect, as claimed by the opponents of surgery, since neither the patients nor the surgeon was anticipating such a result.[1-3] It would have been totally imprudent to ignore such a report by two independent patients. It was, therefore, sensible to design a study to investigate this connection. Thus, a retrospective study was conducted to determine whether there was an association between the removal of the corrugator supercilii muscle and the elimination or significant improvement of MH.[4] Questionnaires were sent to 314 consecutive patients who had undergone corrugator super-cilii muscle resection through endoscopic, transpalpebral, or open forehead rejuvenation procedures. The patients were queried as to whether they had a history of MH before the surgery and, if so, whether the headaches significantly improved or disappeared after surgery. If the answer was affirmative, then the patients were further questioned about the duration of the improvement or cessation of the headaches and the relationship to the timing of the surgery. After an initial evaluation of the completed questionnaires, a telephone interview was conducted to confirm the initial answers and to obtain further information necessary to ensure that the patients had a proper diagnosis of MH based on the International Headache Society criteria.

Of the 314 patients, 265 (84.4%) either responded to the questionnaire or were interviewed, or both. Of this group, 16 patients were excluded because of the provision of insufficient information to meet the International Headache Society criteria, the presence of organic problems, and other exclusions mandated by study design. Thirty-nine (15.7%) of the remaining 249 patients had MH that fulfilled the society criteria. Thirty-one of the 39 (79.5%) with preoperative migraine noted elimination or significant (>50%) improvement in MH immediately after surgery ($p < 0.0001$), and the benefits lasted over a mean follow-up period of 47 months. When the respondents with a positive history of MH were further divided, 16 patients ($p < 0.0001$; McNemar) noticed improvement over a mean follow-up period of 47 months, and 15 ($p < 0.0001$; McNemar) experienced total elimination of their MH over a mean follow-up period of 46.5 months. When divided by MH type, 29 patients (74%) had nonaura MH. Of these patients, the headaches disappeared in 11 patients, improved in 13 patients, and did not change in 5 patients ($p < 0.0001$). Ten patients experienced aura-type headaches, which disappeared or improved in 7 of the patients and did not change in 3 of the patients ($p < 0.0001$). This study suggested for the first time that there is indeed a strong correlation between forehead rejuvenation and potentially removal of the corrugator supercilii muscle and the elimination or significant improvement of MH. However, being a retrospective study, the results were open to criticism. This study offered additional compelling evidence against the placebo effect being the reason for the improvement or elimination of MH after surgery since these patients did not undergo surgery for treatment of MH nor were they aware of such a connection between their surgeries and MH.

Intrigued by the findings from this study, we designed a prospective pilot study investigating the role of corrugator resection and removal of the zygomaticotemporal branch of the trigeminal nerve in MH on a small group of patients ($n = 29$ [24 women, and 5 men], with an average age of 44.9 years [range: 24–63 years]).[5] The patients completed a comprehensive MH questionnaire. The research team neurologist evaluated the patients with moderate to severe MH to confirm the diagnosis using the criteria set forth by the International Headache Society. The team's plastic surgeon injected 12.5 units of botulinum toxin A (BT-A) into each corrugator supercilii muscle group. The patients were asked to maintain an accurate log of their MH and to complete a monthly questionnaire documenting pertinent information related to their headaches. Patients who observed complete elimination of the MH following injection of BT-A underwent resection of the corrugator supercilii muscle group. Those who experienced only significant improvement and who had temple headaches underwent transection of the zygomaticotemporal branch of the trigeminal nerve with repositioning of the temple soft tissues, in addition to removal of the corrugator supercilii

muscles. Once again, patients kept a detailed postoperative record of their headaches.

Twenty-four of 29 patients (82.8%; $p < 0.001$) reported a positive response to the injection of BT-A, 16 (55.2%; $p < 0.001$) observed complete elimination, 8 (27.6%; $p < 0.04$) experienced significant improvement (at least 50% reduction in intensity or severity), and 5 (17.2%) did not notice a significant change in their MH. Twenty-two of the 24 patients who had a favorable response to the injection of BT-A underwent surgery, and 21 (95.5%; $p < 0.001$) observed a postoperative improvement. Ten patients (45.5%; $p < 0.01$) reported elimination of MH and 11 patients (50.0%; $p < 0.004$) noted a considerable improvement. For the entire surgical group, the average intensity of the MH reduced from 8.9 to 4.1 on an analogue scale of 1 to 10, and the frequency of MH changed from an average of 5.2 per month to an average of 0.8 per month. For the group who only experienced an improvement, the intensity fell from 9.0 to 7.5 and the frequency was reduced from 5.6 to 1.0 per month. Only one patient (4.5%) did not notice any change. The follow-up ranged from 222 to 494 days, the average being 347 days.

This study confirmed the potential value of surgical treatment of MH since as many as 21 of 22 patients benefited significantly from the surgery. It was also evident that injection of BT-A is an extremely reliable predictor of surgical outcome. This study further confirmed our findings from the retrospective study. However, being a pilot study, it needed further validation since it did not include a control group. The study also raised the question as to why all of the patients did not respond to surgery if the surgery was indeed the answer. Furthermore, now that the connection was seemingly strong, it was time to start exploring the rationale behind the efficacy of the surgical treatment of MH.

It was about this time that research indicated the role of BT-A in treatment of MH.[6] Based on the findings from the use of BT-A and preliminary surgical findings, we suspected that the elimination of the muscle function was the reason for these surprising positive findings. Additionally, after carefully listening to the patients who had undergone surgery, it became clear that most of these patients who had observed incomplete or partial elimination of MH had pain in the sites other than those that were the target of the surgery such as the occipital region and the retrobulbar area. Anatomical study of these sites seemed to be the next logical step.

Our investigation related to the anatomy of the greater occipital nerve (GON) revealed some enthralling findings.[7] The objective of this study was to determine the GON course, conceivable anatomic variations, and potential sites of entrapment or compression. Twenty fresh cadaver heads were dissected to trace the course of the GON from where the occipital nerve penetrates the semispinalis muscle. It was discovered that the nerve travels through the thickness of the muscle on every specimen. Standardized measurements were used on 14 specimens to determine the location of the emergence of the nerve using the midline and occipital protuberance as landmarks. The point of emergence of the GON from the semispinalis muscle was determined to be centered approximately 3 cm below the occipital protuberance and 1.5 cm lateral to the midline.

As we were completing this anatomical study, a patient who had undergone septorhinoplasty reported that his MH had disappeared. Searching for a potential connection in the literature, we came across an article from Switzerland demonstrating that indeed this surgery had been performed for MH and improved or eliminated MH on many patients.[8] In this study, 299 patients with various types of headaches, including migraine, cluster, and so-called idiopathic headaches, were operated on between 1973 and 1991. Septal correction, resection of the middle concha, ethmoidectomy, and sphenoidectomy on the corresponding headache side or occasionally on both sides were carried out. Most patients (235; 78.5%) were totally asymptomatic postoperatively; 34 (11.5%) had a sensation of pressure in the head on rare occasions but no further migraines, and 30 (11%) continued to experience headaches that occurred only rarely and were mild and of short duration.

Up to this point, the prevailing theory behind MH pathogenesis included four basic concepts: (1) neuronal hyperexcitability during the interictal phase; (2) cortical spreading depression (CSD) as the basis of aura; (3) trigeminal nerve activation at a peripheral and central origin that accounts for the headache; and (4) the provocative concept that progressive central sensitization is possibly related to periaqueductal gray matter damage. Of these four concepts, our findings supported peripheral activation of the trigeminal nerve. MH is postulated to be caused by dilatation of large vessels innervated by the trigeminal nerve. Vasodilatation is the consequence of release of calcitonin gene–related peptide, substance P, and neurokinin A found in the cell bodies of trigeminal neurons. What prompts the release of these peptides remains unclear. We proposed that it may be the mechanical stimulation of the potentially hyperexcited, peripheral sensory nerves that instigates the cascade of events. In fact, in 3 out of 4 trigger sites that we studied, the sensory nerves traverse the muscles. As to the fourth site, contact between the turbinates and the deviated septum may cause MH in some patients.

More knowledge about the anatomy of the zygomaticotemporal branch of the trigeminal nerve seemed in order at this time. A study was conducted to determine the site of emergence of this nerve from the deep temporal fascia and to identify the number of its accessory branches and their locations. An initial pilot study, conducted on 20 patients, concluded that the main zygomaticotemporal branch emerges from the deep temporal fascia at a point on average 17 mm lateral and 6 mm cephalad to the lateral palpebral commissure, commonly referred to as the lateral canthus. These measurements, however, were obtained after dissection of the temporal area, rendering the findings less reliable. Another study included 20 consecutive patients, 19 women and 1 man, between the ages of 26 and 85 years, with an average age of 47.6 years.[9] Those who had a history of previous trauma or surgery in the temple area were excluded. Before the start of the endoscopic forehead procedure, the likely topographic site of the zygomaticotemporal branch was marked 17 mm lateral and 6 mm cephalad to the lateral orbital commissure on the basis of the information extrapolated from the pilot study. The surface mark was then transferred to the deeper layers using a 25-gauge needle stained with brilliant green. After endoscopic exposure of the marked site, the distance between the main branch of the trigeminal nerve or its accessory branches and the tattoo mark was measured in posterolateral and cephalocaudal directions. In addition, the number and locations of the accessory branches of the trigeminal nerve were recorded.

On the left side, the average distance of the emergence site of the main zygomaticotemporal branch of the trigeminal nerve from the palpebral fissure was 16.8 mm (range: 12–31 mm) in the posterolateral direction and an average of 6.4 mm (range: 4–11 mm) in the cephalad direction. On the right side, the average measurements for the main branch were 17.1 mm (range: 15–21 mm) in the posterolateral direction and 6.65 mm (range: 5–11 mm) in the cephalic direction. Three types of accessory branches were found in relation to the main branch: (1) accessory branch cephalad, (2) accessory branch lateral, and (3) accessory branches in the immediate vicinity of the main branch. This anatomical information has proven colossally helpful in injection of BT-A in the temporalis muscle to eliminate the trigger sites in the parietotemporal region and surgical management of MHs triggered from this zone.

Armed with the anatomical information and having an understanding that there are at least four common trigger sites, we designed a prospective randomized study.[10] The purpose of this study was to investigate the efficacy and safety of surgical deactivation of MH trigger sites. The study was designed by a team of a board-certified neurologist who was a headache specialist, a biostatistician, and a plastic surgeon. The number of patients in each group and the randomization process were decided by the experienced biostatistician. Of 125 patients diagnosed with MH and selected by the neurologist of the team using the International Headache Society criteria, 100 were randomly assigned to the treatment group and 25 served as controls, with the 4:1 allocation decided by the biostatistician considering our results from the retrospective and prospective pilot studies. Patients in the treatment group were injected with BT-A for identification of trigger sites (not for therapeutic reasons). Eighty-nine patients who noted improvement in their MH for 4 weeks following injection of BT-A underwent surgery. Eighty-two of the 89 patients (92%) in the treatment group who completed the study demonstrated at least 50% reduction in MH frequency, duration, or intensity compared with the baseline data; 31 (35%) reported elimination and 51 (57%) experienced improvement over a mean follow-up period of 396 days. In comparison, 3 of 19 control patients (15.8%) recorded reduction in MH during the 1-year follow-up ($p < 0.001$), and no patients observed elimination. All variables improved significantly for the treatment group when compared with the baseline data and the control group, including the Migraine-Specific Quality of Life questionnaire (MSQ), the Migraine Disability Assessment score (MIDAS), and the Short Form-36 Health Survey (SF-36). The mean annualized cost of migraine care for the treatment group ($925) reduced significantly compared with the baseline expense ($7,612) and the control group ($5,530; $p <0.001$). The mean monthly number of days lost from work for the treatment group (1.2 days) was reduced significantly compared with the baseline data (4.41 days) and the control group (4.4 days; $p < 0.003$).

The common adverse effects related to injection of BT-A included discomfort at the injection site in 27 patients after 227 injections (12%), temple hollowing in 19 of 82 patients (23%), neck weakness in 15 of 55 patients (27%), and eyelid ptosis in 9 patients (10%). The common complications of surgical treatment were temporary forehead and occipital anesthesia on 89 patients (100%) on the operated sites, temporary dryness of the nose in 12 of 62 patients who underwent septum and turbinate surgery (19.4%), rhinorrhea in 11 (17.7%), intense scalp itching in 7 of 80 patients who underwent forehead surgery (8.8%), and minor hair loss in 5 patients (6.3%). Sinus infection was observed in 3 patients (3.4%). After this experience, we altered our postoperative antibiotic course and had patients continue taking antibiotics while their intranasal surgical sites were healing and from thereon, sinus infections have been eliminated. Recurrence of the septal deviation was noted in

12 patients (13.5%), but these were not symptomatic. Intense itching was reported by 7 patients (7.9%). All 10 parameters in validated tools demonstrated measurable and statistical significant improvement in the MSQ, MIDAS, and SF 36.

This study demonstrated that surgical deactivation of migraine trigger sites can eliminate or significantly reduce migraine symptoms effectively and safely. Interestingly, when the results of the surgery within the first 3 postoperative months were compared to the subsequent three quarters, there was a steady, statistically significant pattern of improvement in each quarter. This finding is totally contrary to what one would expect from a placebo effect, where the initial higher success rate would decline over time. Additionally, when the surgical outcome was analyzed independently at each trigger site, there was significant increase in both improvement and elimination rates, which indicated that some of the failures or suboptimal results had to do with the fact that we failed to detect and deactivate all trigger sites in every patient. This has been confirmed with a more recent study.[11]

In a 5-year follow-up arm of the above study,[12] patients were examined by the research team and were asked to complete the MH log, the SF-36, MSQ, and MIDAS questionnaires that they had completed previously, at a minimum of 60 months after surgery. The neurologist and the surgical team were able to follow 79 patients for 5 years. Ten patients who had observed significant improvement but not elimination underwent deactivation of additional (different) trigger sites during the 5-year follow-up period in an attempt to eliminate their headaches. This opens the study to criticism. However, the overall outcome with or without inclusion of these 10 patients was no statistically significant difference. It would have been improper to deny the opportunity for additional improvement in the quality of life for these patients who had agreed to participate in the study merely to prevent criticism.

Sixty-one of 69 (88%) patients continued to have a positive response to the surgery after 5 years ($p < 0.0001$). Twenty (29%) reported complete elimination of MH, 41 (59%) noticed a significant decrease in frequency, severity, and duration of MH, and 8 (11%) observed no significant change ($p < 0.0001$). All of these endpoints were assessed independently. When compared to the baseline values, all 10 measured variables including MIDAS, MSQ, and SF-36 improved significantly at 60 months ($p < 0.0001$), confirming that the achieved positive results were enduring.

To offer the ultimate evidence of the efficacy of surgical decompression of MH trigger sites, we planned a study to include a sham surgery arm with enormous inherent challenges. After obtaining institutional review board (IRB) approval from two separate boards, patients with a single trigger site or MH predominantly emanating from one site were recruited and randomized to receive placebo surgery or real surgery.[13] Two board-certified and fellowship-trained headache specialists selected the patients based on the International Headache Society criteria. The number of subjects assigned to the real surgery and sham surgery groups as well as their randomization technique into the groups was decided by a highly respected and experienced biostatistician. The patients underwent injection of BT-A to simulate the surgery effect by paralyzing the muscle (not for therapeutic reasons). The patients in the sham surgery group underwent the incision and the nerves and muscles were identified, but the muscles were not touched and the nerves were not decompressed.

Like any other study completed in our center, all data were collected and stored by the study nurse coordinator without any input from the surgical team and delivered directly to the biostatistician of the team. The data were analyzed and the results section of the article was written by the biostatistician who also prepared the tables and graphs without any input from the surgical team.

Seventy-five of 76 patients enrolled in the study completed the 1-year follow-up. Forty-nine of those patients served in the treatment group and 26 were assigned to the sham surgery group. Forty-one of the 49 (83%) patients benefitted from the real surgery compared to 15 of 26 (56%) patients in the sham surgery group ($p = 0.014$). While 28 (57%) patients in the real surgery group observed complete elimination, only 1 patient in the sham surgery group reported elimination ($p < 0.0001$).[13]

5.2 Basic Science Study in Support of Peripheral Mechanisms

In a more recent study, the nerves of patients who had MH were compared to those without MH to investigate whether there were any structural differences.[14] Following IRB approval, a segment of the zygomaticotemporal branch of the trigeminal nerve on 15 patients who experienced MH were compared to the nerves of the 15 patients without MH using proteomic analysis and electron microscopy. Two independent departments at Case Western Reserve University (Center for Proteomics and Bioinformatics and Department of Neurosciences) analyzed their study results and the researchers independently wrote the respective results sections concluding that the nerves of patients with MH had myelin deficit. The implications of this study are that patients who suffer from

MH have vulnerable nerves that could be readily irritated peripherally and thus begin the cascade of events that ultimately results in the full MH complex.

Following confirmation that migraine surgery is efficacious and safe and the pathophysiology is myelin deficiency, we focused on ways to improve the outcomes.

5.3 Factors Contributing to Success and Failure

The purpose of this study was to identify factors that contribute to MH surgery failure and success.[15] A retrospective chart review was conducted on patients who underwent surgery for MH and had at least 11 months of follow-up. The study population included three groups: migraine surgery success, improvement, and failure. Thirty-six unique data points were collected for each patient.

A total of 169 patients met the inclusion criteria. Of these, 66 patients comprised the migraine surgery success group (S, complete elimination of MHs); 67 comprised the migraine surgery improvement group (I, >50% reduction in migraine frequency, intensity, or duration); and 36 comprised the migraine surgery failure group (F, <50% reduction in migraine frequency, intensity, or duration). Significant differences among the groups included age at surgery (S > I, $p = 0.02$), migraine frequency (S < I; $p = 0.02$), age of migraine onset (S > I; $p = 0.003$; S >F; $p = 0.04$), history of head or neck injury (S < I; $p = 0.04$), daily use of over-the-counter migraine medications (S < I; $p = 0.05$), visual symptoms (S > I; $p = 0.02$), increased intraoperative bleeding (S < F; $p = 0.04$; I < F; $p = 0.04$), site I (S > F; $p = 0.0006$; I > F; $p = 0.0004$), site II (S > F; $p = 0.015$), single operative site (S < F; $p = 0.005$), one to two operative sites (S < F; $p = 0.04$; I < F; $p = 0.01$), and four operative sites (S > I; $p = 0.05$; S > F; $p = 0.04$). Factors associated with migraine surgery failure include increased intraoperative bleeding and surgery on fewer trigger sites. Factors associated with migraine surgery success are older age of migraine onset, higher rate of visual symptoms versus improvement group, surgery at site I or II, and deactivating all four operative sites.

5.4 Is Injection of Botulinum Toxin A Necessary for Identification of the Trigger Sites?

In another study, the medical charts of 335 migraine surgery patients were reviewed. Patients who received stepwise diagnostic BT-A injections were placed in the treatment group ($n = 245$). Patients who did not receive BT-A were placed in the control group ($n = 90$). The preoperative and 12-month postoperative MH frequency, duration, and intensity were compared to determine the success of the operations.

Seventy-two of 90 control patients (80%) experienced a significant improvement (a decrease of at least 50% in MH frequency, duration, or intensity) at 12 months after surgery, with 29 (32%) reporting complete elimination. Of the 245 patients in the treatment group, 207 (84%) experienced a significant improvement, with 89 (36%) experiencing complete elimination. The surgical success rate of the treatment group was not significantly higher than that of the control group ($p = 0.33$). Although BT- A can be a useful diagnostic tool, this study demonstrated that there was no statistically significant difference between the injection of BT-A and the use of a constellation of symptoms to identify trigger sites.[16]

5.5 Foraminotomy and Frontal Migraine Headaches

Although 92% of patients who underwent surgical decompression of the supraorbital nerve for treatment of frontal MHs through resection of the glabellar muscle group achieved at least 50% improvement, only two-thirds demonstrated complete resolution of symptoms. We investigated the role of additional decompression methods by comparing surgery outcomes between patients who underwent glabellar myectomy alone and patients who also underwent supraorbital foraminotomy.[17]

Outcome measures, including MH frequency, severity, duration, and MH index score, were reviewed retrospectively and analyzed statistically for 43 age-matched patients who underwent glabellar myectomy for release of the supraorbital nerve and 43 patients who underwent glabellar myectomy with supraorbital foraminotomy from 2002 to 2010.

The myectomy group statistically matched the myectomy with foraminotomy group for age, number of surgical sites, and preoperative headache characteristics ($p < 0.05$). For the myectomy and myectomy with foraminotomy groups, postoperative migraine frequency was 7.8 per month versus 4.1 per month, severity was 5.6 versus 4.4, MH index score was 26.5 versus 11.1, and persistent forehead pain was 48.8 versus 25.6%, respectively. These differences were all statistically significant ($p < 0.05$). Duration of headache was unchanged ($p = 0.17$).

We concluded that the supraorbital foramen is a potential site of supraorbital nerve compression that can trigger frontal MH. If it is present, we strongly recommend foraminotomy to ensure complete release of the supraorbital nerve to optimize outcomes. The results also support consideration of release of any fibrous bands across the supraorbital notch.

5.6 Socioeconomic Impact

A study was designed to compare the direct and indirect cost of MH care before and after migraine surgery and to evaluate any postoperative changes in patient participation in daily activities.[18]

Eighty-nine patients enrolled in a migraine surgery clinical trial completed the MSQ, the MIDAS questionnaire, and a financial cost report preoperatively and 5 years postoperatively.

Mean follow-up was 63 months (range: 56.9–72.6 months). Migraine medication expenses were reduced by a median of $1,997.26 annually. Median cost reduction for alternative treatment expenses was $450 annually. Patients had a median of three fewer annual primary care visits for the MH treatment, resulting in a median cost reduction of $320 annually. Patients missed a median of 8.5 fewer days of work or childcare annually postoperatively, with a median regained income of $1,525. The median total cost spent on MH treatment was $5,820 per year preoperatively, declining to $900 per year postoperatively. Total median cost reduction was $3,949.70 per year postoperatively. The mean surgical cost was $8,378. Significant improvements were demonstrated in all aspects of the MSQ and MIDAS questionnaires.

This study illustrates that surgical treatment is a cost-effective care, reducing direct and indirect costs. Patients may also expect improvements in the performance and increased participation in activities of daily living.

5.7 Endoscopic versus Transpalpebral Frontal Migraine Headache

This study was designed to compare the efficacy of the transpalpebral versus endoscopic approach to decompression of the supraorbital and supratrochlear nerves in patients with frontal MH.[19]

The medical charts of 253 patients who underwent surgery for frontal MH were reviewed. These patients underwent either transpalpebral nerve decompression ($n = 62$) or endoscopic nerve decompression ($n = 191$). Minimum 12-month postoperative migraine frequency, duration, and intensity were analyzed to determine the success of the surgeries.

Forty-nine of 62 patients (79%) in the transpalpebral nerve decompression group and 170 of 191 patients (89%) who underwent endoscopic nerve decompression experienced a successful outcome (at least 50% decrease in migraine frequency, duration, or intensity) after 1 year from surgery. Endoscopic nerve decompression had a statistically significantly higher success rate than transpalpebral nerve decompression ($p < 0.05$). Thirty-two patients (52%) in the transpalpebral nerve decompression group and 128 patients (67%) who underwent endoscopic nerve decompression observed elimination of MH. The elimination rate was significantly higher in the endoscopic nerve decompression group than in the transpalpebral nerve decompression group ($p < 0.03$). The inferior success rate of the transpalpebral approach could be attributed to not routinely searching for a foramen either preoperatively using the perinasal sinus CT (computed tomography) or intraoperatively by direct exploration, something that is part of the frontal migraine surgery protocol today.

5.8 Botox Is Prognosticator for Success of Surgery

A study was conducted to determine whether botulinum BT-A injections can serve as a prognosticator for migraine surgery success.[20] Patients who underwent migraine surgery from 2000 to 2010 were reviewed. Patients were included if they had BT-A injection before surgery, and had completed post-injection, 1 year post-surgery MH questionnaires. Outcome variables include patient demographics, migraine frequency, severity, duration, and MH index. Treatment success was defined as at least 50% reduction in MH index.

One hundred eighty-eight patients were included; 144 reported successful MH reduction after BT-A injection (success group) and 44 did not (failure group). The groups were well matched for age, MH characteristics, and number of surgical sites ($p < 0.05$). The surgery success rate was significantly higher in the BT-A group overall (90.3% vs. 72.3; $p \leq 0.003$). The success rate was even higher when the surgery site–specific symptoms were only considered (97.9% vs. 71.4%; $p \leq 0.0001$), rather than over all MH. BT-A success was prognostic for surgery success at the frontal trigger site (trigger site I; 92.5% vs. 69.2%; $p < 0.012$), the temporal trigger site (trigger site II; 95.5% vs. 73.3%; $p < 0.005$), and the occipital trigger site (trigger site IV; 95.9% vs. 62.5%; $p < 0.0003$). Six patients had exclusively septum or turbinate (site III) surgery, and all failed injections.

Positive botulinum toxin type A response is a significant predictor of migraine surgery success. When injections fail, nonmuscular abnormalities

should be considered. However, use of BT-A is not practical on every case and we have demonstrated the constellation of symptoms could be used as effectively for detection of the trigger sites.

5.9 Role of Third Occipital Nerve in Treatment of Occipital MH

The third occipital nerve is often encountered during the occipital migraine surgery; however, its contribution to MHs is unclear. The objective of this study was to determine whether removing the third occipital nerve plays any role in the clinical outcomes of occipital migraine surgery.[21] A retrospective comparative review was conducted on all occipital MH (site IV) patients from 2000 to 2010. Inclusion criteria were (1) completion of migraine questionnaire, (2) migraine site IV decompression, and (3) minimum 6 months of follow-up. Patients were divided into those who had the third occipital nerve removed and those who did not. Outcome variables included overall MH index reduction and site IV pain elimination. A total of 229 patients met the study inclusion criteria. The third occipital nerve was removed in 111 patients and it was not removed in 118 patients. These two groups were comparable in terms of age, gender, and number of surgical sites, and were statistically well matched regarding preoperative headache characteristics. MH index reduced 63% for the group in which the third occipital was removed compared to 64% reduction in the group in which the nerve was not removed. Patients who underwent third occipital removal experienced 26% elimination compared to 29% elimination on the group in which the third occipital nerve was not removed ($p = 0.45$). The surgery success with at least 50% reduction in MH was 80% for the group who had the third occipital nerve removed compared to 81% success rate on the group in which the third occipital nerve was not removed. There was also no difference between the two groups in symptomatic neuroma formation. Site IV–specific MH elimination was similar between the two groups (58% for the group in which the nerve was removed vs. 64% for the group in which the nerve was not removed). We concluded that removal of the third occipital nerve did not alter migraine surgery success. However, it is important to note that the nerve was removed only if it was visualized.

5.10 Preoperative Narcotic Use and Surgery Outcomes

This study focused on the impact of preoperative narcotic medication use on outcomes of surgical treatment of MH.[22] A retrospective comparative review was conducted with patients who had undergone migraine surgery. Data gathered included demographic information, baseline MH symptoms, migraine surgery sites, postoperative MH characteristics 1 year or more following surgery, and preoperative migraine medication use. Patients were grouped based on preoperative narcotic medication use. The narcotic users were subdivided into low and high narcotic user groups. Preoperative migraine characteristics were comparable between groups and the outcomes of migraine surgery were compared between the groups.

Outcomes in 90 narcotic users were compared with those for 112 patients who did not use narcotic medications preoperatively. Narcotic users showed statistically significantly less reduction in frequency, severity, and duration of MHs after surgery. Narcotic users had clinical improvement in 66.7% of patients and elimination in 18.9% versus 86.6 and 36.6%, respectively, in the nonnarcotic group. The group that consumed narcotics had significantly lower rates of improvement in all migraine indices.

Previous studies have discouraged the routine use of narcotic medications in the management of migraine medications. This study demonstrated that narcotic medication use before MH surgery may predispose patients to worse outcomes postoperatively. Because pain cannot be objectively documented, the question remains of whether this failure to improve the pain was indeed a suboptimal response to surgery or the need for narcotic substances related to the dependency.

5.11 Preoperative Migraine Headache Frequency and Surgical Outcomes

It was unknown how migraine frequency influences outcomes. In this study, 488 patients prospectively completed the MH questionnaires preoperatively and at least 11 months postoperatively.[23] Patients were grouped into three cohorts based on migraine frequency of 1 to 14 per month (episodic), 15 to 29 per month (chronic), or those who had MH every day (daily). Statistics were performed with paired t-tests, linear regression, and analysis of variance with Tukey's honestly significant difference test.

All groups experienced a significant benefit from surgery in terms of frequency, duration, and severity of MH, and MH index. Patients experienced significantly different final outcomes based on their frequency cohort with respect to duration ($p = 0.02$), frequency ($p < 0.0001$), and MH index ($p < 0.0001$). However, when the preoperative score is controlled

for, the only significant difference between cohorts occurred in MH index among daily migraineurs compared with episodic ($p = 0.0003$) and chronic ($p = 0.0008$) migraineurs. No other significant findings persisted.

All cohorts, regardless of their frequency of MH, achieved significant improvement in frequency, duration, severity, and MH index. The groups also achieved statistically different final outcomes, but no group benefitted more than the other when improvement is quantified, and patients can expect similar proportional improvement.

5.12 Use of Doppler to Confirm Migraine Headache Trigger Sites

We discovered that the ultrasound Doppler could be used as a tool for identifying the site of irritation of a nerve by an adjacent artery in different migraine trigger sites. A study was designed to assess the correlation between the most intense pain site identified by the patients, presence of ultrasound Doppler signal, and the intraoperative finding of an artery in the target site.[24]

This was a retrospective review of the charts of patients who underwent surgical treatment of MHs involving the auriculotemporal nerve. The target area was identified by asking patients to point to the most intense headache site and most tender area at the time of examination using the index finger tip. This site was marked and the ultrasound Doppler was used to identify the vascular signal. The ultrasound Doppler examination results, intraoperative presence of the superficial temporal artery or its branches, and the involved nerve were recorded and tabulated.

A positive Doppler signal over the area of most intense temporal pain, identified by the patient preoperatively, correlated with intraoperative presence of the artery in 100% of the patients. Doppler signal was noted in 34 sites and arterectomy was carried out in all 34 sites. The results demonstrated that Doppler signal in the site of most intense pain can predictably confirm the presence of an artery in the most painful site and lead to precise location of the nerve irritation by a vessel and thus successful removal of the offending artery.

5.13 Prospective Comparison of Two Temporal MH Deactivation Techniques

We compared the reduction of MH frequency, days, severity, and duration after surgical decompression versus avulsion of the zygomaticotemporal branch of the trigeminal nerve for treatment of temporal MH.[25]

Twenty patients with bilateral temporal MH were randomized to undergo avulsion of the zygomaticotemporal branch of the trigeminal nerve on one side and decompression via fasciotomy and removal of the zygomaticotemporal artery on the other side. Results were analyzed after a minimum of 12 months of follow-up.

Nineteen patients completed the study. The patients experienced greater than 50% improvement in frequency, migraine days, severity, and duration in 34 of the 38 operative sites (89%). Complete elimination of symptoms was noted in 21 of the 38 operative sites (55%). In the decompression group, migraine frequency was reduced from 14.6 to 2.2 per month, migraine days from 14.1 to 2.3, severity from 7.0 to 2.9, duration from 9.6 to 4.8 hours, and MH index score from 42 to 2.9. In the neurectomy group, frequency decreased from 14.2 to 1.9 per month, migraine days from 14.1 to 2.3, severity from 6.8 to 2.6, migraine duration from 10.1 to 5.3 hours, and the MH index score from 41 to 2.5. There was no statistical significance in reduced MH frequency, days, severity, and duration between the two groups.

We concluded that neurectomy and decompression of the zygomaticotemporal branch of the trigeminal nerve are both appropriate treatment for temporal MH. If decompression fails to provide sufficient relief, neurectomy would offer a second option.

5.14 Retrospective Review of Surgery on Adolescent Population

The purpose of this study was to review outcomes following migraine surgery in an adolescent population.[26] A retrospective review of all patients who underwent surgery from 2000 to 2014 was performed. All patients aged 18 years or younger with at least 1 year of follow-up after surgery were included. Preoperative and postoperative migraine frequency, duration, severity, and MH days and migraine index were analyzed for statistical significance.

A total of 14 patients who underwent 15 operations were analyzed. After an average follow-up of 38.2 months, the frequency of MH per 30-day period was reduced from 25 to 5 ($p < 0.0001$), the MH index decreased from 148.1 to 12.4 ($p < 0.0001$), the duration of headaches (number of hours per 24 hours) declined from 0.71 to 0.25 ($p = 0.002$), severity of headaches diminished from 8.2 to 4.3 ($p = 0.0004$), and migraine days per month declined from 25 to 5 ($p < 0.0001$). Five patients remained free of any symptoms following surgery. One patient had no improvement in frequency of headaches, but did have improvement in severity and duration of headaches. No postoperative complications were noted in this group of patients.

In the adolescent population with MH refractory to traditional medical management, migraine surgery may offer symptomatic improvement of MH frequency, duration, and severity in patients with identifiable anatomical trigger sites. Since some childhood MHs may subside during adulthood, it is crucial to investigate the MH in the siblings, which is a reliable indicator of persistence of MH.

5.15 Current Means for Detection of Migraine Headache Trigger Site

Our 15-year experience with migraine surgery led us to believe that the most common reasons for incomplete response are failure to detect all of the trigger sites or, on rare occasions, inadequate surgery on the trigger sites. Thus, accurate identification of trigger sites is essential. The purpose of this study was to share the authors' current stepwise algorithm for accurately detecting the migraine trigger sites, which has evolved through surgery on nearly 1,000 patients.[27] To begin with, a thorough history is taken. Each patient's constellation of symptoms can point toward one or multiple trigger points. The patient is asked to point to the most frequent site from which MHs originate with one fingertip, and then the site is explored with an ultrasound Doppler. If an arterial Doppler signal is identified at the site, it is considered an active arterial trigger site. Response to a nerve block with a local anesthetic in a patient with an active MH confirms the presence of a trigger site. If the patient does not have pain at the time of the office visit, an injection of BT-A at the suspected trigger site may be considered. Although positive responses to BT-A and nerve block are very helpful and reliable in confirming the trigger sites, negative responses must be interpreted with extreme caution. In patients with an MH starting from the retrobulbar site, a CT scan of the paranasal sinuses is obtained to look for contact points and other pathology that would confirm rhinogenic trigger sites.

5.16 Lesser and Third Occipital Nerves

There is a subset of patients who undergo chemodenervation or surgical release of the GON and note improvement or elimination of the symptoms along the GON course but who experience an emergence of MH symptoms laterally. The authors propose the lesser occipital nerve as the source of pain in those who experience headaches laterally and involvement of the third occipital nerve in those who notice residual symptoms in the midportion of the occipital region.

To test this hypothesis anatomically, 20 cadaver heads were dissected to trace the course of the lesser occipital nerve and third occipital nerve and define the location of these nerves with respect to external landmarks.[28] The midline and a line drawn between the inferior most points of the external auditory canals were used to obtain standardized measurements of these nerves. The location of emergence of the lesser occipital nerve was determined to be an area centered 65.4 ± 11.6 mm from midline and 53.3 ± 15.6 mm below the line between the external auditory canals. The third occipital nerve was found 13.2 ± 5.3 mm from midline and 62.0 ± 20.0 mm down from the line between the two external auditory canals. This information can be used to conduct clinical trials of chemodenervation of these nerves in an attempt to eliminate migraine symptoms in the subset of patients who continue to experience residual symptoms after surgical release of the GON.

5.17 Auriculotemporal Nerve

The auriculotemporal nerve has been identified as one of the peripheral trigger sites for MH. However, its distal course is poorly mapped following emergence from the parotid gland. In addition, a reliable anatomical landmark for locating the potential compression points along the course of the nerve during surgery has not been sufficiently described.

Twenty hemifaces on 10 fresh cadavers were dissected to trace the course of the auriculotemporal nerve from the inferior border of the zygomatic arch to its termination in the temporal scalp.[29] The compression points were mapped and the distances were measured from the most anterosuperior point of the external auditory meatus, which was used as a fixed anatomical landmark.

Three potential compression points along the course of the auriculotemporal nerve were identified. Compression points 1 and 2 corresponded to preauricular fascial bands. Compression point 1 was centered 13.1 ± 5.9 mm anterior and 5.0 ± 7.0 mm superior to the most anterosuperior point of the external auditory meatus, whereas compression point 2 was centered at 11.9 ± 6.0 mm anterior and 17.2 ± 10.4 mm superior to the most anterosuperior point of the external auditory meatus. A significant relationship was found between the auriculotemporal nerve and superficial temporal artery (compression point 3) in 80% of hemifaces, with three patterns of interaction: a single site of artery crossing over the nerve (62.5%), a helical intertwining relationship (18.8%) and nerve crossing

over the artery (18.8%). Findings from this cadaver study provide information relevant to the operative localization of potential compression points along the auriculotemporal nerve.

5.18 Anatomical Variations of Greater Occipital Nerve

A study was conducted to elucidate anatomical variations of the GON and surrounding occipital tissues.[30] Anatomical and surgical variations were prospectively recorded for 272 patients who underwent GON decompression by a single surgeon between 2003 and 2012. Data collection was performed intraoperatively and specifically for the purposes of this study. Documented anatomical variations of the GON and surrounding occipital region included the extension of trapezius musculature to the midline, abnormal lymph nodes, and GON branching. Variations in the surgical procedure were also noted, including resection of a lateral portion of semispinalis capitis muscle and occipital arterectomy.

The GON pierced the semispinalis muscle in all patients bilaterally. The extension of trapezius musculature to the midline was discovered in 67.3% of patients and lymph node enlargement was discovered in 1.5% of patients. Branching of the GON was noted in 7.4% of patients and muscles or vessels between GON branches were noted in 3.7% of patients. Occipital arterectomy was required in 64.0% of patients and resection of a lateral segment of semispinalis muscle was required in 10.7% of patients.

The new anatomical variations described in this study improve understanding of the intraoperative anatomy of the occipital region and prevent difficulty in finding the GON due to dissection in the wrong plane, ensuring that MH patients receive maximal benefit from surgical treatment.

5.19 Conclusion

Through retrospective, prospective pilot, prospective randomized, prospective randomized sham surgery, and 5-year follow-up, we have demonstrated the efficacy, longevity, and safety of surgical treatment of MHs. The clinical studies were all IRB approved and included at least one board-certified neurologist specializing in headaches who diagnosed and selected the patients based on the International Headache Society criteria and ruled on conditions such medication overuse headaches. The studies were designed by the entire team but mostly by an experienced biostatistician. The data were collected by the nurse coordinator without the involvement of the surgical team and submitted directly to the biostatistician for analysis of the data who wrote the results section of the articles.

References

[1] Mathew PG. A critical evaluation of migraine trigger site deactivation surgery. Headache 2014;54(1):142–152

[2] Diener HC, Bingel U. Surgical treatment for migraine: time to fight against the knife. Cephalalgia 2015;35(6):465–468

[3] McGeeney BE. Migraine trigger site surgery is all placebo. Headache 2015;55(10):1461–1463

[4] Guyuron B, Varghai A, Michelow BJ, Thomas T, Davis J. Corrugator supercilii muscle resection and migraine headaches. Plast Reconstr Surg 2000;106(2):429–434, discussion 435–437

[5] Guyuron B, Tucker T, Davis J. Surgical treatment of migraine headaches. Plast Reconstr Surg 2002;109(7):2183–2189

[6] Binder WJ, Brin MF, Blitzer A, Schoenrock LD, Pogoda JM. Botulinum toxin type A (BOTOX) for treatment of migraine headaches: an open-label study. Otolaryngol Head Neck Surg 2000;123(6):669–676

[7] Mosser SW, Guyuron B, Janis JE, Rohrich RJ. The anatomy of the greater occipital nerve: implications for the etiology of migraine headaches. Plast Reconstr Surg 2004;113(2):693–697, discussion 698–700

[8] Novak VJ, Makek M. Pathogenesis and surgical treatment of migraine and neurovascular headaches with rhinogenic trigger. Head Neck 1992;14(6):467–472

[9] Totonchi A, Pashmini N, Guyuron B. The zygomaticotemporal branch of the trigeminal nerve: an anatomical study. Plast Reconstr Surg 2005;115(1):273–277

[10] Guyuron B, Kriegler JS, Davis J, Amini SB. Comprehensive surgical treatment of migraine headaches. Plast Reconstr Surg 2005;115(1):1–9

[11] Punjabi A, Brown M, Guyuron B. Emergence of Secondary Trigger Sites after Primary Migraine Surgery. Plast Reconstr Surg 2016;137(4):712e–716e

[12] Guyuron B, Kriegler JS, Davis J, Amini SB. Five-year outcome of surgical treatment of migraine headaches. Plast Reconstr Surg 2011;127(2):603–608

[13] Guyuron B, Reed D, Kriegler JS, Davis J, Pashmini N, Amini S. A placebo-controlled surgical trial of the treatment of migraine headaches. Plast Reconstr Surg 2009;124(2):461–468

[14] Guyuron B, Yohannes E, Miller R, Chim H, Reed D, Chance MR. Electron microscopic and proteomic comparison of terminal branches of the trigeminal nerve in patients with and without migraine headaches. Plast Reconstr Surg 2014;134(5):796e–805e

[15] Larson K, Lee M, Davis J, Guyuron B. Factors contributing to migraine headache surgery failure and success. Plast Reconstr Surg 2011;128(5):1069–1075

[16] Liu MT, Armijo BS, Guyuron B. A comparison of outcome of surgical treatment of migraine headaches using a constellation of symptoms versus botulinum toxin type A to identify the trigger sites. Plast Reconstr Surg 2012;129(2):413–419

[17] Chepla KJ, Oh E, Guyuron B. Clinical outcomes following supraorbital foraminotomy for treatment of frontal migraine headache. Plast Reconstr Surg 2012;129(4):656e–662e

[18] Faber C, Garcia RM, Davis J, Guyuron B. A socioeconomic analysis of surgical treatment of migraine headaches. Plast Reconstr Surg 2012;129(4):871–877

[19] Liu MT, Chim H, Guyuron B. Outcome comparison of endoscopic and transpalpebral decompression for treatment of frontal migraine headaches. Plast Reconstr Surg 2012;129(5):1113–1119

[20] Lee M, Monson MA, Liu MT, Reed D, Guyuron B. Positive botulinum toxin type a response is a prognosticator for migraine surgery success. Plast Reconstr Surg 2013;131(4):751–757

[21] Lee M, Lineberry K, Reed D, Guyuron B. The role of the third occipital nerve in surgical treatment of occipital migraine headaches. J Plast Reconstr Aesthet Surg 2013;66(10):1335–1339

[22] Adenuga P, Brown M, Reed D, Guyuron B. Impact of preoperative narcotic use on outcomes in migraine surgery. Plast Reconstr Surg 2014;134(1):113–119

[23] Molavi S, Zwiebel S, Gittleman H, Alleyne B, Guyuron B. The effect of preoperative migraine headache frequency on surgical outcomes. Plast Reconstr Surg 2014;134(6):1306–1311

[24] Guyuron B, Riazi H, Long T, Wirtz E. Use of a Doppler signal to confirm migraine headache trigger sites. Plast Reconstr Surg 2015;135(4):1109–1112

[25] Guyuron B, Harvey D, Reed D. A prospective randomized outcomes comparison of two temple migraine trigger site deactivation techniques. Plast Reconstr Surg 2015;136(1):159–165

[26] Guyuron B, Lineberry K, Nahabet EH. A retrospective review of the outcomes of migraine surgery in the adolescent population. Plast Reconstr Surg 2015;135(6):1700–1705

[27] Guyuron B, Nahabet E, Khansa I, Reed D, Janis JE. The current means for detection of migraine headache trigger sites. Plast Reconstr Surg 2015;136(4):860–867

[28] Dash KS, Janis JE, Guyuron B. The lesser and third occipital nerves and migraine headaches. Plast Reconstr Surg 2005;115(6):1752–1758, discussion 1759–1760

[29] Chim H, Okada HC, Brown MS, et al. The auriculotemporal nerve in etiology of migraine headaches: compression points and anatomical variations. Plast Reconstr Surg 2012;130(2):336–341

[30] Junewicz A, Katira K, Guyuron B. Intraoperative anatomical variations during greater occipital nerve decompression. J Plast Reconstr Aesthet Surg 2013;66(10):1340–1345

6 Detection of Migraine Headache Trigger Sites

Bahman Guyuron

Salient Points

- The patient is asked to keep a 1 month log of migraine headaches (MHs) recording the MH starting site, frequency, intensity, duration and the associated symptoms prior to the first visit.

- During the first visit, the patient is asked to identify the most common and most intense MH sites which are confirmed by reviewing the log.

- The constellation of symptoms related to each trigger site is reviewed to further validate the MH beginning site.

- The patient is asked to point to the area of the most pain or tenderness using the tip of the index finger, especially if the patient is experiencing headaches at the time of examination.

- If the patient can identify a specific site that is tender, it is marked and a Doppler signal is searched for.

- A combination of the patient identifying the site of onset of MH, presence of site-specific constellation of symptoms and presence of a Doppler signal at the site of inception of pain or most tender point reliably identify the trigger site.

- Elimination of pain after a nerve block with injection of 0.5 to 1 mL of ropivacaine (Naropin) in the identified or suspected trigger site can further confirm the trigger site.

- Should the patient fail to identify the trigger site as a specific point and refer to a diffuse zone of active pain, the potentially involved nerve in that anatomical zone is blocked with injection 0.5 to 1 mL of ropivacaine (Naropin), if the patient has pain at the time of examination.

- If the patient refers to a zone of inactive pain at the time of examination and is unable to identify a point of pain or tenderness, one must either rely on the constellation of symptoms or inject botulinum toxin A (BT-A), unless the headache starts from a retrobulbar site.

- A paranasal computed tomography (CT) scan can be invaluable in assessing the MHs originating from the retrobulbar site.

- The constellation of symptoms including retrobulbar pain, CT findings of contact points, concha bullosa, paradoxical curl, and/or Haller's cell are diagnostic of rhinogenic trigger site.

- A negative nerve block or lack of response to BT-A injection does not necessarily exclude MH in the suspected site since central sensitization and diffuse inflammation of the trigeminal nerve or the occipital nerve may prevent a meaningful response to a nerve block or injection of BT-A.

- Injection of BT-A may not be effective on sites where MHs are the consequence of irritation of the nerve by intranasal contact points, a vessel, fascial band, or within a bony foramen.

- It is essential to make sure the patients understand that while most will have complete elimination of migraine headache, for some, additional surgeries could be necessary to achieve a migraine-free state.

- For the ease of communication, the migraine trigger sites have been assigned Latin numbers from I to VII.

6.1 Introduction

Our substantial experience with migraine surgery has led us to the conclusion that the patients who experience incomplete response to the initial surgery often observe migraine headaches (MHs) arising from a site that was not detected during assessment for the initial surgery. While the patients may surmise that the surgery failed, often after further inquiry, they concur that the residual MHs are not emanating from the initial surgery sites. Most commonly, these are secondary MH trigger sites.[1] However, on rare occasions, the failure to respond is the consequence of incomplete primary surgery. Paying careful attention to the patients' statements has helped us to improve our trigger site detection techniques over the last 17 years. In this chapter, we will review our current means of detection of the migraine trigger sites in detail (▶ Fig. 6.1).

6.2 Maintenance of Migraine Log

The patients are asked to keep a 1-month log of MHs while they are waiting to be seen. The logging period does not necessarily have to be exactly 1 month, but a 30-day log would offer the most valuable information. The goal of this log is to document the common trigger sites from which the MHs initiate, the intensity, frequency, and duration of MHs, and to assemble the symptoms associated with the MHs. These findings can then be compared to postoperative values. This logging technique avoids solely relying on patient recall. Most patients with MH are on a variety of medications that impair their memory and cognitive function and thus may not be able to accurately remember the information that is essential for detection of the trigger sites and the decision about the surgery site and overall patient candidacy for surgical treatment of MHs. This log will also document the associated symptoms and medications they consume each time they experience MH.

6.3 Identifying Migraine Starting Point

The most valuable piece of information that the patient can provide to the examiner is the site of onset

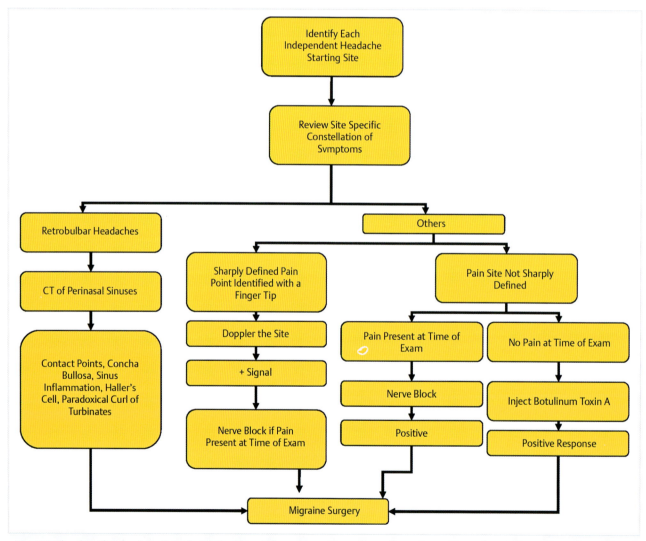

Fig. 6.1 The algorithm for detection of migraine trigger sites.

of MHs. On the initial assessment of headache sites, the patients are often very vague about the migraine site and point to the area with the whole hand or with multiple fingers. It is paramount to elicit as much cooperation from the patient and to identify the trigger site as narrowly as possible. To that end, it is important to encourage the patient to use the index fingertip and point to the area where they may experience beginning of the pain or tenderness several times to assure consistency. Often the patients may resist the idea of having a point of pain or tenderness, but after emphasizing the importance of this information, one can almost invariably produce the intended results from the examination. Each patient may have multiple trigger sites and the initial step is to focus on the point from which the MHs commence most commonly and are most severe. After confidently detecting the most common trigger site, the next question will center on the second most common trigger site the MH arises independent of the first trigger site. Extension of pain from one site to another area is very common and it does not constitute a second trigger site. Through a step-by-step process and with persistence, one can identify each autonomous trigger site. The identified site is then marked lightly with a marker. There are rare patients who, despite perseverance, may not be able to identify a point of origin for their MH. Asking this group of patients to obtain a photograph while they are pointing to the area of the pain at the onset of MH in different times could prove very helpful. Again, it is extremely important to assure by repeated questioning that the observed MH in each site is an independent headache site, it is not the extension of the ache from another site, and headache can be present in each site without the other sites being painful.

6.4 Constellation of Symptoms

After the patient points to the area of pain, it is helpful to consider the constellation of symptoms that the patient is experiencing. Again, the most important piece of information that the patient can supply the examiner is the site of origin of the MH. However, the constellation of symptoms that aid in the detection of trigger sites is also very useful in confirming the triggers sites, especially on patients who cannot precisely identify the point of inception of headaches. The common collection of symptoms for all four main trigger sites is listed in ▶ Tables 6.1–6.4. This assemblage of symptoms is extremely reliable and often aids in the discovery of trigger sites, even in the absence of Doppler signal or failure of patient to point to the precise site of start of MH. However, the more information one garners, the more likely that all trigger sites will

Table 6.1 Constellation of symptoms related to the frontal migraine headache (MH)

The pain starts at the eyebrow level or immediately below or above it

Doppler signal is often present in the most tender sites

There is strong corrugator muscle activity causing deep frown lines on animation and repose

The points of emergence of the supraorbital and supratrochlear nerves from corrugator muscle or the foramen are tender to the touch

Patients commonly have eyelid ptosis on the affected side at the time of active pain

Pressure on these sites may abort the MH during the initial stages

Application of cold or warm compresses on these sites often reduces or stops the pain

The pain is usually imploding in nature

Stress can often result in triggering MH

Table 6.2 Constellation of symptoms related to the temporal migraine headache (MH)

The pain starts in the temple area about 17 mm lateral and 6.5 mm cephalad to the lateral canthus

Patients usually wake up in the morning with pain having been clenching or grinding their teeth all night

Often the pain is associated with tenderness of the temporalis or masseteric muscle

One may see wearing of the dental facets

Rubbing or pressing the exit point of the zygomaticotemporal branch of the trigeminal nerve from the deep temporal fascia can stop or reduce the pain in the beginning

Application of cold or warm compresses to this point may reduce or stop the pain

The pain is characterized as imploding

Stress can trigger MH in this site

Doppler signal could be identified in this site

Table 6.3 Constellation of symptoms related to the rhinogenic migraine headache (MH)

The pain starts behind the eye

Patient commonly wakes up with the pain in the morning or at night

Commonly the MHs are triggered by weather changes

Rhinorrhea can accompany the pain on the affected side

This type of MH can be related to nasal allergy episodes

Menstrual cycles can trigger MH

The pain is usually described as exploding

Concha bullosa, septal deviation with contact between the turbinates and the septum, septa bullosa, and Haller's cell can be seen in the computed tomography

Table 6.4 Constellation of symptoms related to the occipital migraine headache (MH)

The pain starts at the point of exit of the greater occipital nerve from the semispinalis capitis muscle (3.5 cm caudal to the occipital tuberosity and 1.5 cm off the midline)

Doppler signal could be identified in the most tender spot

The patients may have a history of whiplash injury

The neck muscles are usually tight

Heavy exercise can trigger MH

Compression of this site can stop the pain in the early stage, while at the later stage, this point is tender

Application of cold or heat at this site may result in some improvement in the pain

Stress can be a major trigger for the occipital MH

be detected and dealt with, resulting in a successful elimination of the MH, rather than improvement.

It is vital to realize that many of the symptoms can be shared between different trigger sites. Also, the pain from one site can extend to another site. It is of utmost importance to keep redirecting the patient's attention to the origin of the pain and confirm the independence of the identified site.

Some findings are highly specific, such as pain starting from the eyebrow area with a prominent corrugator supercilii muscle group on patients with frontal MHs. Patients with temporal MHs arising from irritation of the zygomaticotemporal branch of the trigeminal nerve (ZTBTN) point to the hollowed area in the temple centered about 17 mm lateral and 6.5 mm cephalad to the lateral canthus. Pain lateral or posterior to this site could be related to the posterior branch of this nerve, or anterior branch of the auriculotemporal nerve, or even a branch of the zygomaticfacial nerve. Patients with zygomticotermporal nerve trigger site commonly report nightly tooth grinding or clenching and wake up in the morning with pain in this site. Patients with rhinogenic trigger sites will have pain starting from behind the eyes, almost always associated with weather changes, and commonly wake up in the middle of night or in the morning with headaches. Orgasm- or menstrual-related MHs are commonly experienced in this site. It is interesting to note that all of these conditions that trigger rhinogenic MHs cause enlargement of the turbinates through hormonal, atmospheric, or postural changes. The increase in the size of the turbinates may intensify the contact between the structures inside the nose. Occipital MHs related to the greater occipital nerve commonly begin close to the midline or within 5 cm of the midline of the occipital region, at least 2.5 cm above the occipital hairline and extend more cephalically in a vertical and lateral fashion.

The lesser occipital MHs are closer to the hairline and more lateral to the greater occipital nerve territory, and often extend to the top of the ear or temple. The patients with occipital MH or neuralgia commonly have a history of whiplash injury.

6.5 Using the Fingertip

One of the most important aspects of detecting the trigger site is successful solicitation of patient cooperation in pointing to the headache commencement site with a fingertip. This could prove extremely easy in some patients and very challenging in others. It is crucial to be relentless. Repeated questioning could help in identifying and confirming this site. It is possible to entice even patients who do not have pain at the time of examination to find a tender point that is the likely site of the beginning of the MH. Another way to find this spot is to ask the patient to point to the site where they or their spouse or friends press on firmly to abort or mitigate the headache in the beginning of the migraine cascade. Pressure in the spot stops the blood flow through the vessel near the nerve that could be causing irritation of the nerve. Not every patient will reliably find this spot, but the overwhelming majority will do so. When the trigger site is identified, it is lightly marked to be explored with a Doppler probe.

6.6 Doppler Signal

One of the tools that have become exceptionally helpful in the detection of trigger sites is the ultrasound Doppler. We have discovered that patients who point to the MH site, especially those with nummular headaches, almost invariably have a Doppler signal at that site.[2] It is fascinating that this signal can be so consistently identified if the patient can point to the migraine site precisely. Sometimes it is necessary to ask the patient to point to the area several times before detecting the Doppler signal. However, this Doppler signal can be commonly identified on the first attempt. Our anatomical dissections[3-12] have demonstrated that, frequently, there is a vessel that is crossing the nerve or is intertwined with the nerve that is often the site of the start of MHs. The nerve/vessel interaction as the mechanism of peripheral irritation has been the subject of previous reports going back many decades.[13] Our electron microscopy and proteomic study has demonstrated that patients with MH have a myelin deficiency.[14] Whether this pulsation in the vessel next to a myelin-deficient nerve is the real trigger source of MH needs to be proven, but it seems to be a logical potential explanation.

To use the Doppler accurately, the patient is asked to point to the area of pain beginning with the index fingertip. The site is marked and the Doppler is utilized to detect a signal. It may be necessary to move the Doppler probe around to small extent to identify the vessel signal. A combination of the pain starting at a specific site that the patient can point to with an index finger and detection of a Doppler signal at that site is an extremely reliable and objective means of identifying the trigger site. The ultrasound Doppler is a handheld, low-cost device that has become an integral part of our migraine surgery practice for several years.

Our team has demonstrated that the auriculotemporal nerve intersects the superficial temporal artery in approximately 34% of examined specimens.[15] While in most cases this is a single point crossover, this could also be a helical intertwining of the vessel with the nerve, although the latter relationship is more common with the occipital nerve than with the auriculotemporal nerve. The lesser occipital nerve can also cross over or under the occipital artery branches 55% of the time through a simple intersection.[3] This crossover point can be commonly found 16 to 22 mm caudal to the external auditory canal and 51 mm lateral to the midline.

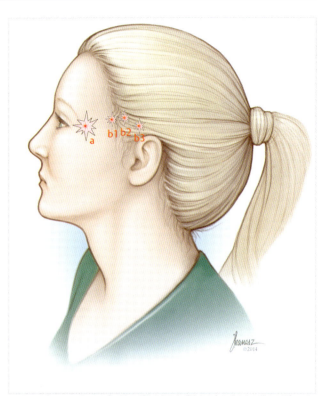

Fig. 6.3 Artistic rendering of variety of temple trigger sites. The ZTBTR nerve (a) and branches of the auriculotemporal nerves where often the temporal trigger sites can extend from lateral to the ZTBTN (zygomaticotemporal branch of the trigeminal nerve) sites to directly above the ear helix (b1, b2, b3).

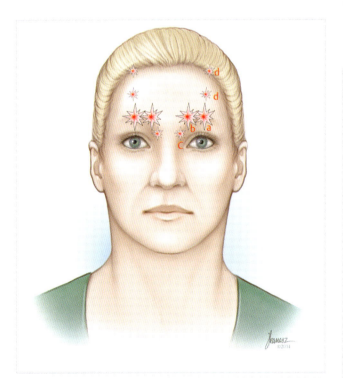

Fig. 6.2 Artistic illustrations of common and rare frontal trigger sites including supraorbital (a), supratrochlear (b), caudal branch of the supratrochlear (c), and distal branch or supraorbital (d; possible nummular headache site).

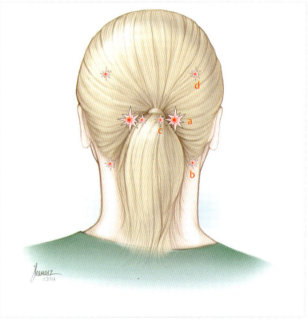

Fig. 6.4 Illustration of the greater occipital (a), lessor occipital (b), the third occipital trigger sites (c), and some nummular or distal greater occipital trigger sites (d).

The ultrasound Doppler has also been an extremely valuable tool in identifying a secondary trigger site following decompression of the main trigger sites. These sites are along the course of the previously decompressed nerve but are often more peripheral than the main trigger sites, such as the vertex, upper forehead, lateral upper cervical area, and especially the temporal area. These commonly behave like nummular headaches. The site of the detectable temple trigger ultrasound Doppler signal could be at any point from near the origin of the ZTBTN to the area immediately above the ear and sometimes in the preauricular region (▶ Figs. 6.2–6.4). It is intriguing to see how often one can find a Doppler signal on these rare MH trigger sites.

6.7 Nerve Block

On patients who refer to the pain area as a zone rather than a point or on those who have a detectable Doppler signal, one can further confirm the trigger sites with a nerve block, so long as the patient has pain at the time of examination. The patient is asked to point to the site of pain and the area is marked and infiltrated with 0.5- to 2-mL ropivacaine (Naropin) depending on the trigger site and the depth where the nerve is located. Most of the time, an injection of 0.5 to 1 mL is sufficient. A 30- or 31-gauge needle with a length of 0.5 to 1 inch is used depending on the site. The preauricular temporal, lesser occipital, supraorbital, and supratrochlear MH sites are injected with a 0.5-inch needle, while the occipital and ZTBTN sites may have to be injected with a 1-inch needle and requires 1 to 2 mL. Almost invariably, the patients will experience improvement or elimination within a few minutes (maximum of 5 to 10 minutes). While a positive response to the nerve block is highly reliable and confirms the presence of a trigger site, a negative response does not rule out the contribution of that site to MH. When the entire trigeminal tree is inflamed and there is central sensitization, it would not allow the local anesthetic to eliminate the pain completely. In this regard, likening the trigeminal nerve to a tree and the tree catching on fire is a particularly helpful analogy for the patients. Explain that if a tree branch catches on fire and one immediately pours water on that branch, one can avoid extension of the fire to the other branches and the fire will be extinguished. When the entire tree is on fire, however, it is hard to ascertain from where the fire started and even if it is detected and water poured on that branch, it is not going to save the entire tree. Our goal, like in the tree-and-fire example, is to identify the branch that is the initial trigger site to stop the process before the cascade of events results in the entire side or even both sides of the head becoming painful.

This explanation helps the patients better understand the nature of the condition and the prodigious role that finding the site of onset of the MH plays in the management of the headaches and why a nerve block may not be effective and it loses its diagnostic value if the blocking agent is injected late.

For the patients who have zonal pain rather than a site that is identified with the index finger, one must block the nerves that could possibly be irritated such as the supraorbital, supratrochlear, the main auriculotemporal, or the greater occipital nerve.

Occasionally, the patients have pain in rare sites such as the infratrochlear, zygomaticofacial, radix, and the terminal branches of main nerves. Almost invariably, one can identify a Doppler signal in those sites as well.

6.8 Botulinum Toxin A

Botulinum toxin A (BT-A) was an integral part of our trigger detection process during our initial studies on migraine surgery. However, we gradually came to the conclusion that adherence to our algorithm, while applicable for local patients, was extremely cumbersome and sometimes impractical for the patients who resided a long distance from our clinic. Additionally, we noted that the patients who could possibly benefit from surgery were denied this treatment due to failure to respond to BT-A. This injection may produce a positive change on several trigger sites such as when the pain originates from a rhinogenic trigger site or when there is vascular or mechanical irritation of the nerves without muscle involvement. Furthermore, the process became too costly since often the insurance companies would not cover the injection of BT-A for detection of trigger sites. Moreover, we compared the outcome of migraine surgery on patients with or without detection of trigger sites using BT-A in a study and came to the conclusion that there was no statistical difference.[16] Considering these facts, we now rarely use BT-A as a means to discover the trigger sites. However, for those surgeons who are inexperienced, this could be a useful means of confirming the trigger sites. For the patients who would choose to have BT-A injection and reside far from the our clinic, all of the independent trigger sites are first identified using the 1-month log and the constellation of symptoms, and the sites are injected with BT-A. On patients who have frontal MH, we use 25 units of BT-A dissolved in 0.5 cc for bilateral injection of the glabella muscles (each side will be injected 12.5 units). Similarly, 25 units of BT-A dissolved in 0.5 mL is injected in each temporalis muscle for temporal MH. The same amount of BT-A is injected at the greater occipital site bilaterally. Again, all of these sites could be injected in one visit as long as they are identified as independent trigger sites. The results will be checked 1 month later and each independent site is evaluated separately. The follow-up assessment is done through Skype, FaceTime, or by phone for the long-distance patients. For local patients, one may choose to either inject all of the independent sites in one visit or in a staged fashion. With a phased injection protocol, the most common trigger site is first injected with BT-A. The patient is examined after 1 month to assess the results. The injection will be repeated in the second most common MH site, should the headaches not be eliminated. This process will be repeated until all of the trigger sites are detected. Generally, the trigger sites can be identified with a maximum of three injections.

It is important to realize that BT-A may not be effective on the trigger sites where the irritation is related to rhinogenic sources, a vessel, fascial band, or bony tunnel like the supraorbital nerve that passes through the supraorbital foramen.[17,18] It is for this reason that a negative response to BT-A has to be interpreted cautiously. Sometimes, the intensity of the headaches is reduced after injection of BT-A beyond the trigger sites because it reduces the additional insult related to the muscle movement or as a consequence of the anti-inflammatory effects of BT-A. The frequency, however, seldom changes. We have demonstrated that a positive response to BT-A increases the success rate.[19] Although this study result on the surface may seem to be in contrary to our study comparing the constellation of symptoms as described earlier, in reality they are not contradictory. One is predicting the role of the BT-A response on overall outcome, while the other one is comparing the results of the surgery when BT-A is used for detection of the trigger sites as opposed to the constellation of symptoms.

6.9 Use of Computed Tomography Scan

For the patients who have MH starting from the retrobulbar area, use of a computed tomography (CT) scan is an exceedingly reliable tool. The presence of any contact points between the septum and the turbinates or the septum and the lateral wall of the nose, concha bullosa, paradoxical curl of the turbinates, Haller's cell, and any sinus inflammation could trigger MH.[20] These are the patients who commonly have the constellation of symptoms outlined in ▶ Table 6.3, the most important one being pain starting from behind the eyes and especially weather changes. Additionally, the same CT scan can be used for identification of a supraorbital fora-

Table 6.5 Classification of the trigger sites

Site I Frontal Headaches

Site II Temporal Headaches

Site III Rhinogenic Headaches

Site IV Greater Occipital Headaches

Site V Auriculotemporal Headaches

Site VI Lesser Occipital Headaches

Site VII Isolated Sites and Nummular Headaches

men when the patient has a combination of retrobulbar and supraorbital pain. We have demonstrated that this paranasal sinus image can reliably demonstrate the presence of a foramen, thus helping with detection of the trigger site and planning the surgery.[21] For the ease of communication, we have developed a classification of migraine headaches that is outlined in ▶ Table 6.5.[22]

6.10 Conclusion

After a patient keeps a log of MH, the locations of the independent headache sites are identified with a combination of the patient pointing to the pain site, review of constellation of symptoms, use of Doppler to find a vascular signal, nerve block as long as the patient has headache at the time of examination, and CT scan of paranasal sinuses. Positive response to the nerve block and injection of BT-A can help in confirming the trigger sites and assuring deactivation of all of the independent trigger sites in most patients. However, the complexity of the BT-A injection process makes its routine use less practical.

References

[1] Punjabi A, Brown M, Guyuron B. Emergence of secondary trigger sites after primary migraine surgery. Plast Reconstr Surg 2016;137(4):712e–716e
[2] Guyuron B, Riazi H, Long T, Wirtz E. Use of a Doppler signal to confirm migraine headache trigger sites. Plast Reconstr Surg 2015;135(4):1109–1112
[3] Lee M, Brown M, Chepla K, et al. An anatomical study of the lesser occipital nerve and its potential compression points: implications for surgical treatment of migraine headaches. Plast Reconstr Surg 2013;132(6):1551–1556
[4] Junewicz A, Katira K, Guyuron B. Intraoperative anatomical variations during greater occipital nerve decompression. J Plast Reconstr Aesthet Surg 2013;66(10):1340–1345
[5] Chim H, Okada HC, Brown MS, et al. The auriculotemporal nerve in etiology of migraine headaches:

compression points and anatomical variations. Plast Reconstr Surg 2012;130(2):336–341

[6] Janis JE, Hatef DA, Ducic I, et al. The anatomy of the greater occipital nerve: Part II. Compression point topography. Plast Reconstr Surg 2010;126(5):1563–1572

[7] Janis JE, Hatef DA, Thakar H, et al. The zygomaticotemporal branch of the trigeminal nerve: part II. Anatomical variations. Plast Reconstr Surg 2010;126(2):435–442

[8] Janis JE, Ghavami A, Lemmon JA, Leedy JE, Guyuron B. The anatomy of the corrugator supercilii muscle: part II. Supraorbital nerve branching patterns. Plast Reconstr Surg 2008;121(1):233–240

[9] Janis JE, Ghavami A, Lemmon JA, Leedy JE, Guyuron B. Anatomy of the corrugator supercilii muscle: part I. Corrugator topography. Plast Reconstr Surg 2007;120(6):1647–1653

[10] Dash KS, Janis JE, Guyuron B. The lesser and third occipital nerves and migraine headaches. Plast Reconstr Surg 2005;115(6):1752–1758, discussion 1759–1760

[11] Totonchi A, Pashmini N, Guyuron B. The zygomaticotemporal branch of the trigeminal nerve: an anatomical study. Plast Reconstr Surg 2005;115(1):273–277

[12] Mosser SW, Guyuron B, Janis JE, Rohrich RJ. The anatomy of the greater occipital nerve: implications for the etiology of migraine headaches. Plast Reconstr Surg 2004;113(2):693–697, discussion 698–700

[13] Murillo CA. Resection of the temporal neurovascular bundle for control of migraine headache. Headache 1968;8(3):112–117

[14] Guyuron B, Yohannes E, Miller R, Chim H, Reed D, Chance MR. Electron microscopic and proteomic comparison of terminal branches of the trigeminal nerve in patients with and without migraine headaches. Plast Reconstr Surg 2014;134(5):796e–805e

[15] Janis JE, Hatef DA, Ducic I, et al. Anatomy of the auriculotemporal nerve: variations in its relationship to the superficial temporal artery and implications for the treatment of migraine headaches. Plast Reconstr Surg 2010;125(5):1422–1428

[16] Liu MT, Armijo BS, Guyuron B. A comparison of outcome of surgical treatment of migraine headaches using a constellation of symptoms versus botulinum toxin type A to identify the trigger sites. Plast Reconstr Surg 2012;129(2):413–419

[17] Janis JE, Hatef DA, Hagan R, et al. Anatomy of the supratrochlear nerve: implications for the surgical treatment of migraine headaches. Plast Reconstr Surg 2013;131(4):743–750

[18] Fallucco M, Janis JE, Hagan RR. The anatomical morphology of the supraorbital notch: clinical relevance to the surgical treatment of migraine headaches. Plast Reconstr Surg 2012;130(6):1227–1233

[19] Lee M, Monson MA, Liu MT, Reed D, Guyuron B. Positive botulinum toxin type a response is a prognosticator for migraine surgery success. Plast Reconstr Surg 2013;131(4):751–757

[20] Behin F, Behin B, Bigal ME, Lipton RB. Surgical treatment of patients with refractory migraine headaches and intranasal contact points. Cephalalgia 2005;25(6):439–443

[21] Pourtaheri N, Chepla K, Guyuron B. The role of perinasal computerized tomography in the surgical management of patients with frontal migraine headaches. Plast Reconstr Surg (submitted)

[22] Forootan NS, Lee M, Guyuron B. Migraine headache trigger site prevalence analysis of 2590 sites in 1010 patients. J of Plast Reconstr Aesthet Surg 2017;70(2):152-158

7 Surgical Treatment of Frontal Migraine Headaches (Site I)

Bahman Guyuron

Salient Points

- Fifty-six percent of patients with migraine headaches (MHs) experience frontal MH.
- The headache-starting site usually corresponds to the anatomical position of the supraorbital and supratrochlear nerves.
- It is of utmost importance to assure that the MHs arising from the forehead are independent and are not an extension of the retrobulbar MH.
- The patients with frontal MHs usually have deep frown lines, may experience tender spots along the course of the related nerves, and often respond to the nerve blocks and injection of botulinum toxin A favorably.
- Computed tomography (CT) scan of the perinasal sinuses may demonstrate the presence of a main or an accessary supraorbital foramen or both.
- On patients with isolated frontal headaches, surgery is often done through a transpalpebral approach.
- On patients with a combination of frontal and temporal MHs, the endoscopic approach is preferred unless the patient has a long forehead or there is male pattern baldness, in which case the temple surgery is performed endoscopically and the frontal surgery is done through the palpebral approach.
- The transpalpebral approach is the workhorse of frontal MH surgery and is done under sedation or general anesthesia.
- The incision is placed in the most caudal supratarsal crease.
- The initial dissection is between the orbicularis and the orbital septum.
- The supraorbital nerve branch exiting the corrugator muscle is identified first.
- The muscle is removed as thoroughly as possible, saving the nerves.
- The nerves are isolated and the concomitant arteries are cauterized and transected.
- The foramen is unroofed with an osteotome or rongeur, if present.
- Fat graft or fat injection is used to replace the removed muscle volume.
- The incision is repaired using 6–0 fast-absorbing catgut.
- The endoscopic approach requires placement of five or six endoscopic access devices.
- The dissection is subperiosteal.
- The muscles are removed as thoroughly as possible with a grasper while these muscles are pushed against the grasper externally with the nondominant index finger.
- The rest of the procedure is carried out similar to the transpalpebral approach.
- Fat is harvested from the area above the zygomatic arch deep to the deep temporal fascia during the combined technique.
- On patients older than 35 years, the soft tissues are pulled laterally and the superficial temporal fascia is suspended from the deep temporal fascia with a single 3–0 PDS suture for each side.

7.1 Introduction

One of the most common migraine headache (MH) trigger sites is the forehead and 56.6% of patients have the frontal area as a component of their migraine complex. The patients may initially describe a diffuse headache over the entire frontal region. However, with examiner persistence, the patients can often identify the areas from where the headaches start more narrowly. This site commonly corresponds to the supratrochlear and supraorbital nerves. It is crucial to assure that the headache experienced in the frontal region is not an extension of a headache arising from the nose, sinus, or temple. Asking the patient if the frontal headaches can be experienced independent of the other trigger sites can elucidate whether the experienced MHs in the forehead area are triggered primarily from the forehead or are the extension of temporal or retrobulbar headaches to the supraorbital and supratrochlear nerves.

The frontal MHs often begin in the afternoon following a stressful day. These headaches commonly spread across the entire forehead. Rarely, the pain can be limited to the deep branches of the supraorbital nerve and could be confined to a small area close to or even within the hairline laterally along the course of this branch or in an isolated spot. Similarly, pinpoint headaches can be experienced by the patients along the course of the supratrochlear nerve. Almost invariably, when these sites are identified by the patient's fingertip, a Doppler signal can be detected on the site.

The patients with diffuse frontal headaches often have strong frowning muscles with deep frown lines in repose, which get deeper with animation. Commonly, one can elicit tenderness in this trigger site. Additionally, a nerve block may produce very meaningful information, should the patient have pain at the time of examination. Many of the patients with frontal MH respond very favorably to the injection of botulinum toxin A.

Computed tomography (CT) scan findings related to this site include the presence of a main or accessory supraorbital foramen, rather than notch, where the patient usually has the most intense headaches. This is commonly the consequence of irritation of the nerve by the supraorbital vessel, triggering the MH cascade. Confinement of the nerve and vessel to a very tight space could account for the high intensity of the headache in this site even if the headaches are arising from another site, along the course of this nerve. The CT scan of the perinasal sinuses could be useful in detecting the foramen, accessary foramen, or both.

7.2 Surgical Technique

Should the patient have isolated frontal MH, which rarely occurs, the surgical procedure can be done through a transpalperbral[1] or endoscopic approach.[2] Even in the presence of combined temporal and frontal MH, the frontal portion of the surgery could still be carried out through an eyelid incision while the zygomaticotemporal branch of the trigeminal nerve is addressed endoscopically. This also offers an opportunity to explore the supraorbital area endoscopically using the temporal ports. Patients with a receding hairline, congenital long forehead, or those with a round and protruding forehead or proptosis would especially be suitable candidates for the transpalpebral approach.

7.2.1 Transpalpebral Deactivation of Frontal Migraine Headaches

This procedure, which I developed initially for rejuvenation of the forehead on patients with optimal eyebrow position and overactive corrugator muscles, has become the workhorse of frontal migraine decompression.[1] The procedure is done under general anesthesia or deep sedation. If a blepharoplasty is being done at the same time, the conventional blepharoplasty is designed. The most caudal crease is marked first. The second incision will incorporate the redundant skin, and these are joined medially and laterally, placing the lateral incision in the crow's feet line. If no blepharoplasty is intended, the incision will be limited to the inner half of the conventional blepharoplasty incision in the most caudal supratarsal crease (▶ Fig. 7.1). The upper eyelid and glabellar areas are generously infiltrated with lidocaine hydrochloride containing 1:100,000 epinephrine. The eyelid skin incision is made and extended through the orbicularis muscle (▶ Fig. 7.2). The orbital septum is retracted caudally and the orbicularis muscle is pulled cephalically. The easily identifiable plane between these two anatomic structures is entered, and the dissection is continued toward the superior orbital rim using the cautery initially (▶ Fig. 7.3). The dissection is continued with a pair of baby Metzenbaum scissors, spreading the tissues parallel to the muscle fibers (▶ Fig. 7.4). While the orbicularis muscle is being elevated anteriorly, the depressor and corrugator supercilii muscles are exposed immediately cephalad to the orbital rim. The depressor supercilii is further dissected medially and laterally (▶ Fig. 7.5). This muscle is removed using the coagulation power of the cautery (▶ Fig. 7.6). There is a consistent large branch of the supraorbital nerve emerging from the corrugator supercilii muscle. The nerve branch is followed deeper in the muscle with a mosquito hemostat (▶ Fig. 7.7). The corrugator supercilii muscle is then lifted to locate the point of entrance of the nerve to the

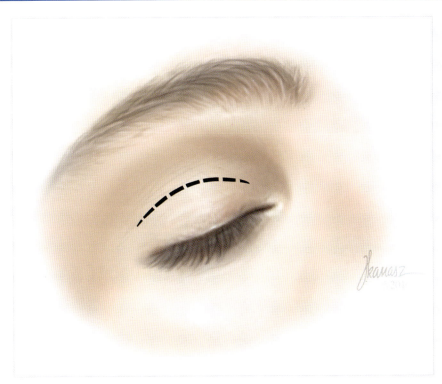

Fig. 7.1 The incision is designed as the inner half of the conventional blepharoplasty incision in the supratarsal crease.

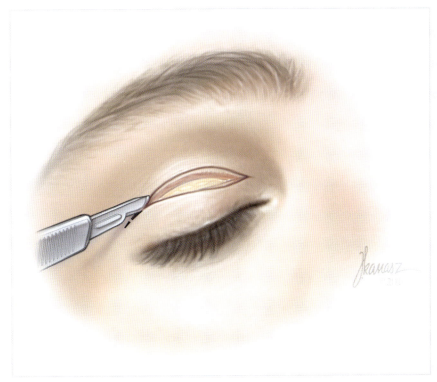

Fig. 7.2 The eyelid skin incision is made and extended through the orbicularis muscle.

muscle (▶Fig. 7.8) and the muscle is removed using the coagulation power of the electrocautery as thoroughly as possible (▶Fig. 7.9). Occasionally, a gentle traction may be sufficient to avulse the muscle, but this should not be a deterring factor in radical removal of the muscle. The lateral fibers of the procerus muscle are also removed conservatively until the supratrochlear nerve is denuded.

Both supratrochlear and supraorbital vessels are removed and the fascia across the supraorbital notch is released, or if there is a supraorbital foramen, it is unroofed with an osteotome or rongeur (▶Fig. 7.10). At this point, a piece of fat is harvested from the medial portion of the upper eyelid, if protruding, and placed into the space created by the resection of the corrugator muscles. The fat

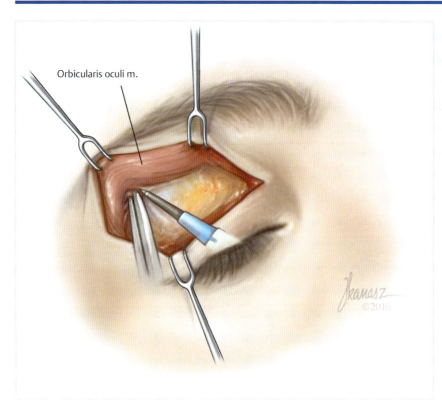

Fig. 7.3 The easily identifiable plane between the orbicularis and orbital septum is entered, and the dissection is continued toward the superior orbital rim using the cautery initially.

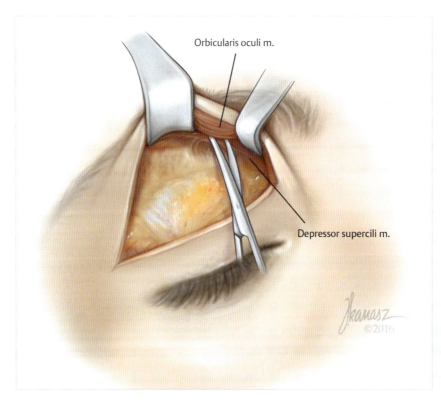

Fig. 7.4 The dissection is continued with a pair of baby Metzenbaum scissors, spreading the tissues parallel to the muscle fibers.

graft is fixed to the underlying periosteum using 6–0 Vicryl or Monocryl to prevent postoperative dislodgement of the fat caudally (▶ Fig. 7.11). The eyelid skin is repaired using 6–0 plain catgut in a running subcuticular fashion, and the incision is treated with bacitracin ointment (see ▶ Video 7.1). Should there not be sufficient amount of fat in the medial compartment of the upper eyelid, 1 cc of fat is aspirated from the abdomen and injected in the muscle site as superficially as possible.

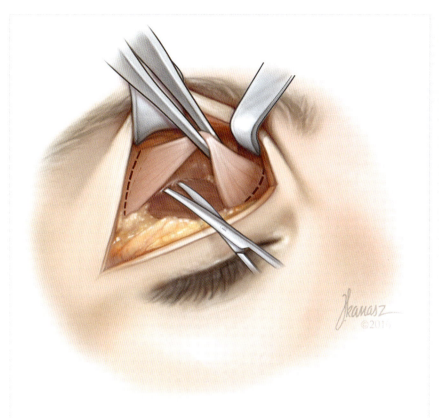

Fig. 7.5 The depressor supercilii muscle is exposed and dissected adequately.

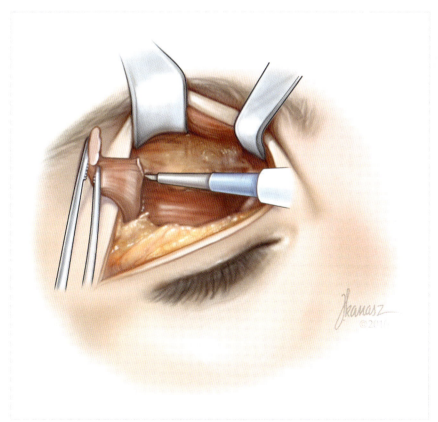

Fig. 7.6 The depressor supercilii muscle is removed using the coagulation power of the electrocautery.

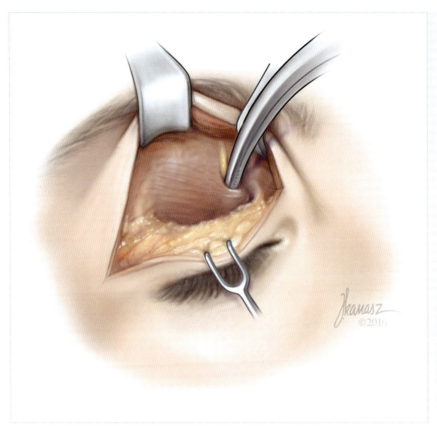

Fig. 7.7 The nerve branch is followed deeper in the muscle with a mosquito hemostat.

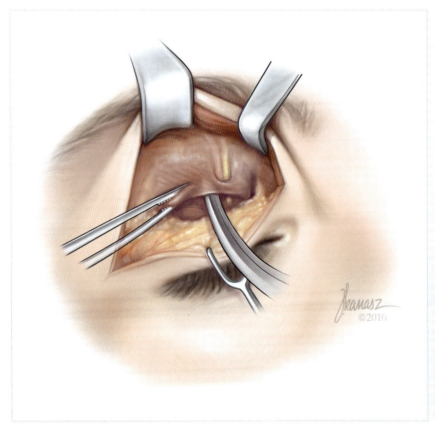

Fig. 7.8 The corrugator supercilii muscle is then lifted to locate the point of entrance of the nerve to the muscle.

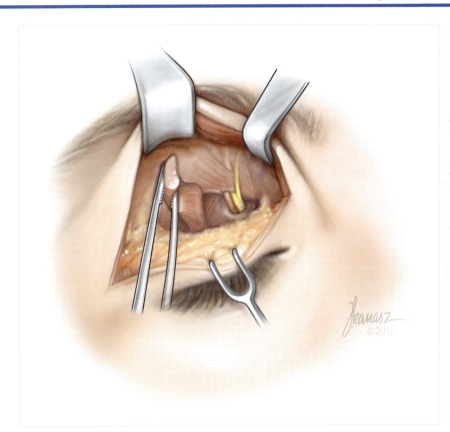

Fig. 7.9 The corrugator muscles and the medial fibers of the procerus muscles are removed as thoroughly as possible using the coagulation power of the electrocautery.

Recovery

Many of these patients have some swelling and bruising around the eyes for 1 week to 10 days. Some swelling may persist for several weeks, but it will be minimal. The patients are instructed to return to light routine activities that are not strenuous soon after surgery, light exercises in 1 week, and full activities in 3 weeks. The sutures are left to dissolve spontaneously, which occurs within a week in most patients. The patients receive intravenous antibiotics during the surgery and for 5 days postoperatively. Bacitracin ophthalmic ointment is used on the incisions for 1 week.

7.2.2 Endoscopic Deactivation of Frontal MH Trigger Sites

This technique is a modification of endoscopic forehead rejuvenation introduced initially by Louis Vasconez and refined by our group.[3] This procedure is completed under general anesthesia or deep sedation. The non-hair-bearing skin of the forehead is injected with Xylocaine containing 1:100,000 epinephrine and the hair-bearing skin is injected with Xylocaine containing 1:200,000 epinephrine. Five ports are commonly used, but patients with a borderline long, round forehead may require the use of two paramedian incisions about 3 to 4 cm apart, totaling six ports. The midline and paramedian incision

sites are marked approximately 0.5 cm behind the hairline. Next, two incisions are marked in the temple area, the first approximately 7 cm and the second 10 cm from the midline only if the patient will have concomitant decompression or removal of the zygomaticotemporal branch of the trigeminal nerve. These incisions are 1.2 to 1.5 cm in length, depending on the thickness of the scalp and subcutaneous tissue. A slightly longer incision is used when the scalp is thick. The hair between these markings is braided by the assistants or gathered in a hemostat on either side of the incision to avoid transfer of hair into the wounds. The entire non-hair-bearing forehead area is injected with lidocaine hydrochloride containing 1:100,000 epinephrine, and the hair-bearing scalp up to approximately 5 cm posterior to the incision is injected with lidocaine containing 1:200,000 epinephrine to minimize the potential for any hair loss. The most lateral incision is made in the right temple area if the temporal surgery is part of the plan (see Video 7.2). This incision is taken through the superficial temporal fascia (STF) down to the deep temporal fascia. Using a pair of baby Metzenbaum scissors and spreading technique, the deep temporal fascia is exposed. Using the Obwegeser periosteal elevator, enough space is created immediately superficial to the deep temporal fascia to allow for insertion of the Endoscopic Access Device (EAD). This silicone device has two shields, one smaller

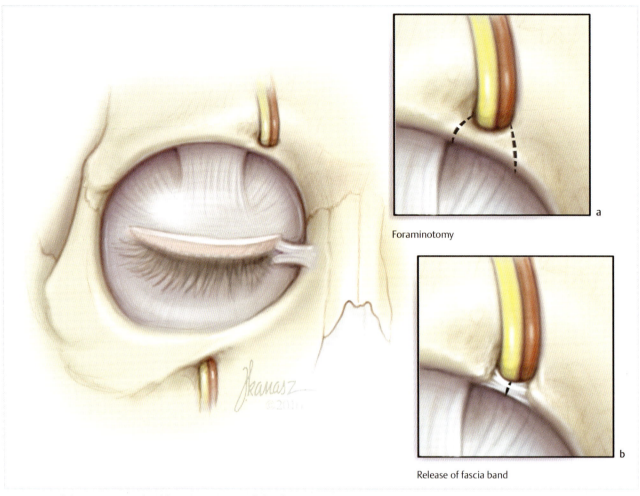

Foraminotomy

a

Release of fascia band

b

Fig. 7.10 If there is a supraorbital foramen, it is unroofed with an osteotome or rongeur.

internal and a larger external, connected by an obliquely oriented tube to properly guide the endoscopic instruments in the target area. To insert, the inner shield of the EAD is folded using a pair of large multi-tooth Adson forceps and while the skin hooks are separating the wound margins, the surgeon introduces the inner shield into the wound step by step, each time trapping the advanced portion of the device with the non-dominant thumb and the index finger. Any resultant fold inside the lumen is easily eliminated by inserting the forceps into the central cannula and running it around the lumen. The periosteal elevator is passed through the first incision and advanced in all directions to dissect the tissues at the plane immediately superficial to the deep temporal fascia in the area surrounding the second incision. Most of the medial dissection will be done under direct vision through the scope. Almost invariably, the second incision falls over the periosteum rather than the temporalis fascia and near the temporal ridge. The second incision is made and extended down to the periosteum. Skin hooks are now placed under the periosteum through the

second incision, and the wound edges are retracted. The second EAD is then introduced in the site. The dissection proceeds medially under the midline incision. At this point, a third incision is made in the midline, and the EAD is again inserted. The procedure is then continued on the left side, starting laterally and advancing medially. The dissected areas are then connected with a periosteal elevator. On patients older than 30 years, the dissection is extended about 3 to 5 cm posteriorly in the subperiosteal plane superficial to the deep temporalis fascia in the temple region to allow for a slight lift at the end of the operation. At this point, the 30-degree 4-mm scope is introduced through the EAD. The dissection is continued toward the supraorbital rim using the endoscope. The arcus marginalis and the periorbita are released along the entire supraorbital rim using a longer curved periosteal elevator. In the temporal area, it is crucial to elevate all of the fat with the STF. The dissection is continued to the zygomatic arch staying on the deep temporal fascia. A rent is made in the deep temporal fascia immediately cephalad to the zygomatic arch as far medially as possible and

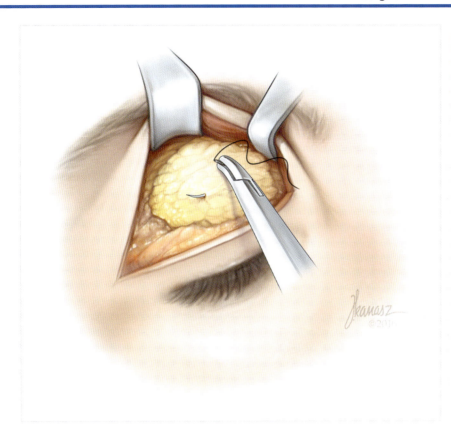

Fig. 7.11 The fat graft harvested from the medial compartment of the upper eyelid is fixed to the underlying periosteum using 6–0 Vicryl or Monocryl to prevent postoperative dislodgement of the fat caudally.

the fat is harvested while pressing on the submalar arch externally. The arcus marginalis is released and the periosteum is elevated over the supraorbital rim until the orbital septum, which has a glistening, grayish appearance, becomes visible. The periosteum along the lateral orbital rim is also released on patients older than 30 years. As the dissection is advanced medially, the supraorbital nerve and vessels become visible, as is the supratrochlear nerve. It is often necessary to remove some or all of the corrugator supercilii muscle to expose the supratrochlear nerve and artery. The supraorbital nerve is closer to the field of dissection and thus more easily identified. The corrugator muscle lies superficial (anterior) to a communicating vein that spans between the supratrochlear and supraorbital veins. This vein is cauterized and the corrugator supercilii, depressor supercilii, and the lateral fibers of the procerus muscles are removed as completely as possible using the Daniel grasper or biopsy forceps. If necessary, the nerves are retracted with a nerve hook for safety. The periosteum over the glabellar area is not transected in almost all patients, unless there is significant medial eyebrow ptosis with skin folding over the radix. The dissection is repeated on the opposite side. The supraorbital and supratrochlear arteries are removed.

If a foramen is encountered, it is converted to a notch using a 2-mm osteotome percutaneously. This requires experience and has to be conducted with utmost care to avoid an injury to the orbital content by those with craniofacial experience. Hemostasis is secured step by step using the Valley Lab suction cautery. The muscle site is then filled with fat, which was harvested from the area above the zygoma earlier. One fascia suspension suture is placed on each side to suspend the anterior portion of the most lateral incision from the deep temporalis fascia. To achieve proper fixation, two single-skin hooks are placed at the junction of the anterior/caudal third and the posterior/cephalad two-thirds of the most lateral incision and the wound edges are retracted. With the surgeon's index finger of the nondominant hand everting the caudal portion of the incision, a 3–0 PDS suture is passed in and out, taking a substantial bite of the STF, which is then passed out/in through the opposite side of the same incision. Next, the skin hooks are placed at the cephalic or posterior third of the incision and are used to retract the scalp as far posteriorly as possible in the direction of the desired vector, usually 45 degrees, on patients older than 30 years to produce slight lift. This vector is predominantly directed laterally and cephalad. The suture that has been passed through the anterior portion of the incision is then passed through the deep temporal fascia. The suture is tied incrementally as the surgeon watches the eyebrow being repositioned to the level deemed aesthetically pleasing. The periosteum and the galea are repaired with 5–0 Monocryl, and the skin is repaired using 5–0 plain catgut. Before the patient is transferred to the recovery room, the forehead area, particularly the area of the supratrochlear and supraorbital nerves, is injected with generous amounts of Naropin to minimize postoperative discomfort.

Recovery

Recovery from the surgery is similar to transpalpebral corrugator resection. However, the magnitude of periorbital swelling could be less. The incisions are covered with a thin layer of bacitracin for about 1 week. The patients are allowed to shower in 2 days and wash the area gently. Use of a hair dryer is prohibited for 2 to 3 weeks. Light activities are resumed soon after surgery, light exercises in 1 week, and full activities in 3 weeks. The patients are encouraged to walk soon after surgery.

7.3 Treatment of Isolated Headache Sites

Some patients have distinct trigger points in the forehead or the anterior scalp after deactivation of migraine trigger sites. These patients can identify the site with their fingertip and commonly volunteer pointing to the site without prompting. A Doppler signal can almost invariably be identified in the site. A nerve block could be highly informative to the surgeon and reassuring to the patients as long as the patient is experiencing headaches at the time of the office visit. For those patients who have isolated sites below the eyebrow and in the supraorbital rim, a transpalpebral incision is used to remove the offending vessel, after confirming its presence with a Doppler. For the peripheral sites located in the midforehead or frontal area, a small (5- to 6-mm-long) incision is made directly over the pain site under local anesthesia after the site is identified by the patient and confirmed with the Doppler signal, nerve block, or both. Injection of lidocaine with 1:100,000 epinephrine will minimize the bleeding. The offending vessel is removed and often there is a strand of the nerve above, below, or crossing the vessel, which is also removed. The incision is repaired using 6–0 Monocryl and 6–0 fast-absorbing catgut. The wound is covered with waterproof dressing and the patient is allowed to return to work the same day or the next day without any limitations.

References

[1] Guyuron B, Michelow BJ, Thomas T. Corrugator supercilii muscle resection through blepharoplasty incision. Plast Reconstr Surg 1995;95(4):691–696
[2] Liu MT, Chim H, Guyuron B. Outcome comparison of endoscopic and transpalpebral decompression for treatment of frontal migraine headaches. Plast Reconstr Surg 2012;129(5):1113–1119
[3] Guyuron B, Michelow BJ. Refinements in endoscopic forehead rejuvenation. Plast Reconstr Surg 1997;100(1):154–160

8 Surgical Treatment of Temporal Migraine Headaches (Site II)

Bahman Guyuron

Salient Points

- It is important to differentiate between the migraine headaches (MHs) arising from the main zygomaticotemporal branch of the trigeminal nerve (ZTBTN) and its branches, and those triggered from the anterior branch of the auriculotemporal nerve.

- The ZTBTN emerges from the deep temporal fascia approximately 16 to 17 mm lateral and 6 mm cephalad to the lateral canthus.

- The surgery could be performed under local or general anesthesia, but the latter is preferred when dealing with the main nerve and the former is better for the MHs arising from the branches of this nerve.

- This surgery is done endoscopically through two radial incisions, 1.5 cm in length and about 3–3.5 cm apart, with the medial/cephalad incision being placed about 7 cm from the frontal hairline midline and the second incision about 10–10.5 cm from the midline.

- The area is infiltrated with lidocaine containing 1:100,000 epinephrine.

- The most lateral/caudal incision is made first, deepened to the deep temporal fascia and then blindly dissected with an Obwegeser periosteal elevator sufficient enough to accommodate the Endoscopic Access Devices (EADs).

- The EADs are placed through these two incisions.

- The dissection is extended medially between any fatty tissues and the deep temporal fascia under direct visualization until the ZTBTN and the associated vessels are exposed. No fat is left on the deep temporal fascia during this dissection to assure the safety of the frontal branch of the trigeminal nerve.

- The nerve is either avulsed gently with a grasper or decompressed by enlarging the fascial opening and cauterization and removal of the concomitant vessels.

- For patients older than 30 years, the tissues are suspended laterally from the deep temporal fascia with a 3–0 PDS suture.

- The incisions are closed using 5–0 Monocryl and 5–0 or 6–0 plain catgut.

8.1 Introduction

Temporal migraine headaches (MHs) can arise from the main zygomaticotemporal branch of the trigeminal nerve (ZTBTN) and its branches, or could be the consequence of irritation of the anterior branches of the auriculotemporal nerve. These variations require totally different management. Thus, the differential diagnosis between the origins of these MHs is crucial. For the surgical treatment of auriculotemporal MH, please refer to Chapter 11.

The ZTBTN-related MHs typically arise from an area centered approximately 16 to 17 mm lateral and 6 mm cephalad to the lateral orbital commissure. Almost invariably, there is a hollowed area that can be detected by palpation at the site where this nerve exits from the deep temporal fascia. The posterolateral branch of this nerve could be irritated by the anterior branches of the superficial temporal artery (Site V), causing headaches in the temple close to the sideburn rather than the area mentioned earlier. Surgical management of these headaches is very different and will be discussed later.

8.2 Surgical Technique

The ZTBTN is approached through two radial incisions, one placed approximately 7 cm from the frontal hairline midline and the other 3.5 cm posterolateral and caudal to the first incision (10–10.5 cm from the midline incision). Each of these incisions will be approximately 1.5 cm long and 0.5 cm behind the sideburn or temporal hairline (▶ Fig 8.1). While this operation can be done under local anesthesia, it is ideally performed under general anesthesia, especially if the intention is to avulse the nerve. After the incisions are designed, the temple is infiltrated with lidocaine containing 1:100,000 epinephrine. The hair is braided or gathered in a hemostat to facilitate the dissection. The incisions are made using a number 15 blade. The dissection is deepened to the deep temporal fascia using a pair of baby Metzenbaum scissors. It is crucial to identify the fascia first. For the beginner, it could prove helpful to make a small rent in the deep temporal fascia and visualize the temporal muscle to ascertain the identity of the deep temporal fascia. Using an Obwegeser periosteal elevator, the dissection is extended around the incision immediately superficial to the deep temporal fascia. The Endoscopic Access Devices (Applied Medical Technology, Cleveland, OH) are inserted to create access for the endoscopic tools and to isolate the wound from scalp hair (▶ Fig. 8.2). The dissection is then continued medially, visualizing the site through the scope (▶ Fig. 8.3). Being in the right plane is crucial to the successful identification

of the ZTBTN and avoidance of injury to the frontal branch of the facial nerve. The dissection is continued medially in the plane immediately superficial to the temporal fascia directed toward the lateral orbital rim where the nerve can be found. For the beginner, it may also be helpful to tattoo, through the surface landmark passing the needle deep enough to reach the temporalis fascia, the point where this nerve commonly emerges from the deep temporal fascia (16–17 mm lateral and 6–7 mm cephalad to the lateral canthus) using methylene blue or brilliant green.[1] One can then find the tattoo mark endoscopically to help locate the nerve. Even leaving the 25-gauge needle that has been passed percutaneously at the site while the dissection is being conducted endoscopically may facilitate finding the ZTBTN. It is important to realize that sometimes this nerve may have two and rarely three branches. It is for this reason that, in our view, surgery on this site through an upper eyelid incision may pose limitations. One has to explore the area sufficiently to assure that there are no additional branches.

After the nerve is identified, the concomitant vessel is isolated and cauterized with a bipolar cautery to avoid thermal damage to the nerve. The nerve can be

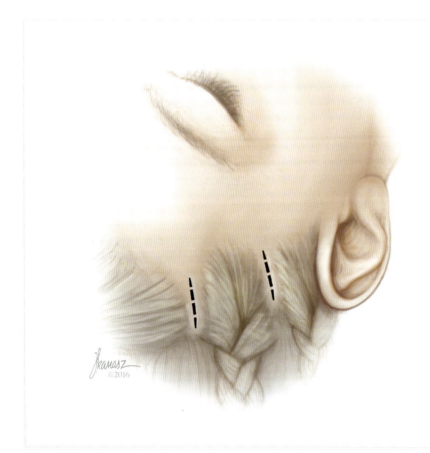

Fig. 8.1 The ZTBTN (zygomaticotemporal branch of the trigeminal nerve) is approached through two radial incisions, one placed approximately 7 cm from the frontal hairline midline and the other 3.5 cm posterolateral and caudal to the first incision (10.5 cm from the midline incision). Each of these incisions will be approximately 1.5 cm long and 0.5 cm behind the sideburn or temporal hairline.

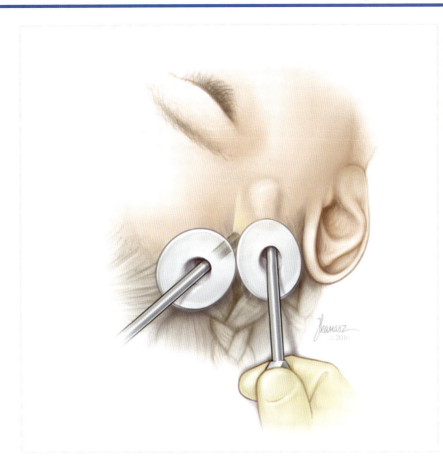

Fig. 8.2 Using an Obwegeser periosteal elevator, the dissection is extended around the incision immediately superficial to the deep temporal fascia. The Endoscopic Access Devices (Applied Medical Technology) are inserted to create access for the endoscopic tools and to isolate the wound from scalp hair.

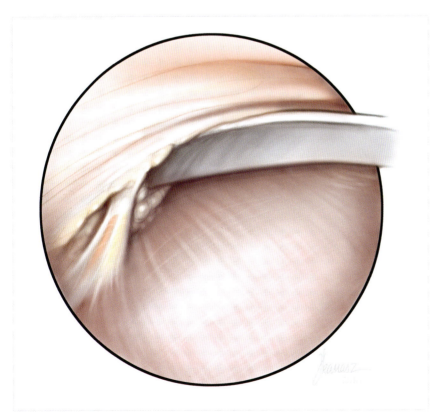

Fig. 8.3 The dissection is then continued medially, visualizing the site through the scope.

treated in one of two ways. It can either be avulsed or decompressed by opening the fascia, especially if there is only a single nerve. The avulsion will be done step by step by grasping the nerve immediately above the deep temporal fascia until the nerve is delivered at least 2–3 cm above the fascia, viewing endoscopically (▶Fig. 8.4). The distal portion of the nerve is then transected at its entrance to the intermediate temporal fascia (distally; ▶Fig. 8.5). Hemostasis is secured and the posterior portion of the deep temporal fascia is explored to make sure there are no other branches.

To decompress the nerve, the deep temporal fascia around the nerve is initially incised with a number 12 blade to enlarge the passage of the nerve (▶Fig. 8.6) and subsequently dilated with a long fine hemostat (▶Fig. 8.7). It is crucial to cauterize and remove any concomitant vessels. Our studies have demonstrated that the avulsion or decompression of the nerve provides equivalent results.[2] If this is the only site that is being operated on, there is no need to harvest fat. However, in combined temporal and frontal MH surgery (Sites I and II), fat is harvested from the area above the zygomatic arch at the junction of this arch and lateral orbital wall by making a rent in the deep temporal fascia.[3] Pressure on the buccal area often facilitates the delivery of fat. The fat is then retrieved step by step. Enough fat is

harvested to replace the removed corrugator muscle. Hemostasis is once more checked.

On patients older than 30 years, the soft tissues are displaced laterally at about a 45-degree angle and a single fascial suspension suture is used to provide slight tightening to the temple area to lift the malar soft tissues, to minimize the potential for the future regrowth and co-optation of the nerve branches and to elevate the lateral eyebrow, especially on patients who have ptotic eyebrows. This suspension is done using 3–0 PDS. To do so, while two single-skin hooks are placed in the medial-caudal portion of the incision, a suture is passed through the most medial-caudal portion of the scalp in an inverted **U** shape starting from the deeper layers, bringing it out, and then passing it out and in through the opposite site of the incision. The suture is then passed through the deep temporal fascia more cephalically and laterally while the skin hooks are repositioned laterally and are retracting the tissues cephalically at a 45-degree angle. The suture is then tightened incrementally until satisfactory lateral repositioning of the eyebrow and the malar soft tissues is achieved. The deeper portion of the incision, including the intermediate fascia, is repaired using 5–0 Monocryl and the skin is repaired using 5–0 or 6–0 plain catgut depending on the density of the hair (see ▶Video 8.1).

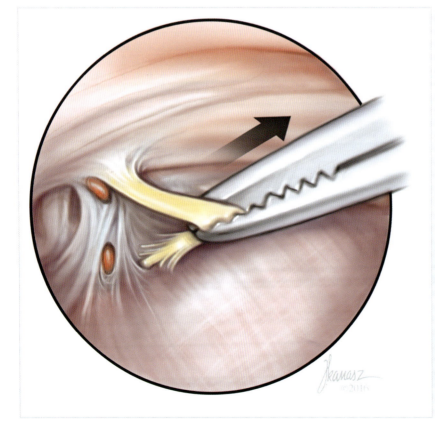

Fig. 8.4 The nerve is then transected at its entrance to the intermediate temporal fascia (distally). Hemostasis is secured and the posterior portion of the deep temporal fascia is explored to make sure there are no other branches.

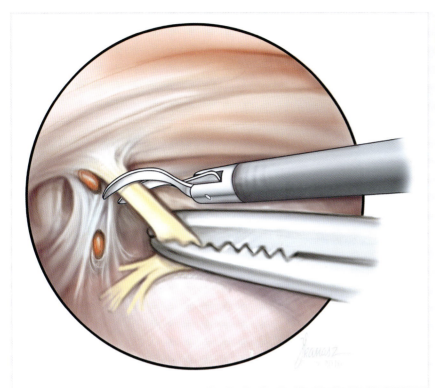

Fig. 8.5 The nerve is then transected at its entrance to the intermediate temporal fascia (distally).

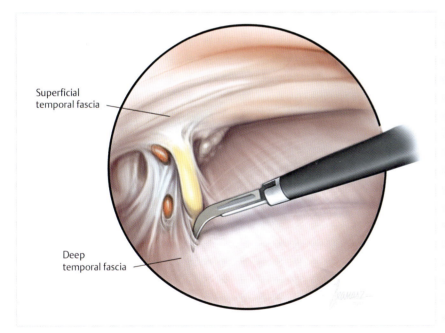

Fig. 8.6 To decompress the nerve, the deep temporal fascia around the nerve is initially incised with a number 12 blade to enlarge the passage of the nerve.

Superficial
temporal fascia

Deep
temporal fascia

8.3 Complications

The potential complications of this operation include injury to the frontal branch of the facial nerve, which is extremely unlikely. If it occurs, it is likely to be temporary. This can be completely avoided by continuing the dissection immediately superficial to the fascia and leaving fat on the fascia. Addition-ally, any cantilever-type movement of the scope which presses the end of the scope on the nerve, damaging the nerve, should be avoided. Another complication of temporal migraine surgery is slight hollowing of the temple area, giving the patients a mild hourglass deformity. Most patients are not aware of this change, but it is something that we have observed.

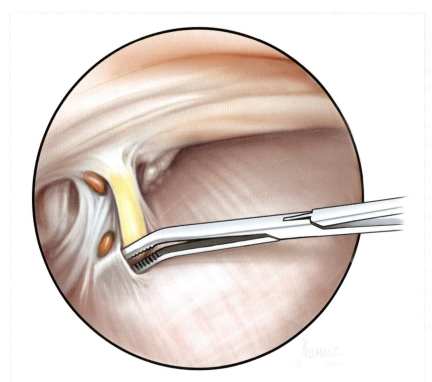

Fig. 8.7 The opening in the fascia is subsequently dilated with a long fine hemostat.

Surgery in this site can truly or ostensibly fail. A true failure, meaning the pain recurs exactly at the same site, is exceedingly rare. The ostensible uncommon failure means the pain seemingly recurs in the same site but with careful investigation it becomes clear that it is a different branch that is involved in this MH. This is due to the secondary triggers at this site often involving the anterior branch of the auriculotemporal nerve and superficial temporal artery.

8.4 Recovery

The recovery from surgery is often extremely smooth. There is usually minimal swelling or there may not be any swelling. The sutures generally dissolve in a week and the patient can resume most social activities in less than a week and vigorous exercises in 2 weeks. Most patients may become symptom free immediately after the surgery. Rarely, the final outcomes may take as long as 3 months. There could be some numbness in the temple area and this is often temporary.

References

[1] Totonchi A, Pashmini N, Guyuron B. The zygomatico-temporal branch of the trigeminal nerve: an anatomical study. Plast Reconstr Surg 2005;115(1):273–277

[2] Guyuron B, Harvey D, Reed D. A prospective randomized outcomes comparison of two temple migraine trigger site deactivation techniques. Plast Reconstr Surg 2015;136(1):159–165

[3] Guyuron B, Rose K. Harvesting fat from the infratemporal fossa. Plast Reconstr Surg 2004;114(1):245–249

9 Surgical Treatment of Rhinogenic Migraine Headaches (Site III)

Bahman Guyuron

Salient Points

- Many of the daily migraine headaches (MHs) have a rhinogenic origin.

- Prolonged supine position, low atmospheric pressure, and hormonal changes can trigger rhinogenic MH.

- Erect position, spraying vasoconstrictors intranasally, and increases in atmospheric pressure can reduce rhinogenic MH.

- The pain is usually behind the eyes and can extend to the temples, forehead, or even occipital areas.

- Computed tomography scan findings may include a large spur touching the turbinates or even the sidewall of the nose, concha bullosa, paradoxical curl of the turbinates, or Haller's cell.

- The surgery is completed under general anesthesia as an outpatient procedure.

- The septoplasty is performed through an L-shaped (Killian) incision, if needed.

- The surgical goal is to eliminate the contact points and decompress the concha bullosa, Haller's cell, or remove the paradoxical curl.

- The deviated portion of the septal cartilage is removed leaving as much of the straight portion of the septal L frame as possible, a minimum of 20 mm anteriorly and 10 mm caudally.

- It is always easier to elevate the posterior portion of the periosteum and extend the dissection anteriorly along the floor on each side of the vomer bone.

- The deviated portion of the vomer bone and the ethmoid plate are removed using a double-action rongeur.

- It is crucial to examine both sides of the nasal cavity thoroughly to assure that the spur and the deviated portion of the septum are removed completely.

- The medial wall of the concha bullosa is removed using a number 4 XPS shaver or with a rongeur.

- The remaining portion of the turbinates is gently cauterized, sprayed with thrombin solution, or both.

- The straight portion of the removed septal cartilage is replaced between the mucoperichondrial layers prior to the repair of the L incision with 5–0 chromic running suture.

- Doyle stents are placed in position and fixed to the membranous septum with 5–0 Prolene suture and kept in place for a minimum of 4 days.

9.1 Introduction

The septum and turbinates are common migraine headache (MH) trigger sites. Frequent occurrence of other headaches arising from this site creates a challenge in differentiating rhinogenic MH and other sinus- and septum-related headaches. Many of the chronic daily MHs with retrobulbar pain emerge from this site. When one considers the anatomical reasons for headaches arising from this trigger site, which is often contact between the septum and the different turbinates, it becomes easy to understand why these patients have daily MH, since the contact is often continuous and thus the headache is relentless.

The patients with rhinogenic MH invariably experience pain behind the eyes, although occasionally it can be felt in the cheek area or even the nasal bones. Commonly, the patients have nausea and vomiting associated with photophobia and phonophobia in addition to the headaches. These symptoms could serve to differentiate MHs from sinus-related headaches. The patients frequently wake up in the middle of the night or in the morning with headaches since prolonged supine position may result in more intense contact sites. The association between atmospheric pressure changes and headaches is so powerful that many of these patients can actually predict the weather changes with impressive accuracy. Additionally, there is a very close connection between rhinogenic MHs and hormonal changes. This is why patients may experience headaches during menstruation. Furthermore, many of the cluster headaches are connected with abnormalities in this site, as we have discussed previously. When one considers the commonality between recumbent position, hormonal and weather changes, and MH, it becomes clear that during all of these conditions, the contact between the turbinates and septum becomes intensified due to enlargement of the turbinates. Some of these patients can ratify that when they stand up or sit up after being awakened by the headaches, the pain can be mitigated. Similar improvement in MH can be noticed when the patient uses nasal decongestants. The explanation is that being in an erect position or use of decongestants reduces the size of the turbinate; thus, the intensity of the contact between the turbinates and the septal spur is diminished, and the headaches often cease or lessen.

The diagnosis is easy with review of the computed tomography (CT) scan images, which provide clear objective evidence. The abnormalities commonly seen in the CT scan include a large spur touching the turbinates or even the sidewall of the nose, concha bullosa, paradoxical curl, or Haller's cell. A small percentage of patients also have chronic sinus disease with thickening of the lining in the sinuses. Reviewing the CT scan with the patients, notwithstanding their medical background, increases the patient's confidence in the surgical plan immeasurably since the patients can easily visualize the abnormalities that are pointed out by the surgeon. The presence of strong symptoms of airway occlusion plays a paramount role in the decision to operate on the septum and the turbinates in patients with insufficient evidence for the nose being an MH trigger site. It is advisable to combine the septoplasty and turbinectomy with deactivation of the other trigger sites in this group of patients with the primary goal being improvement in the airway and the improvement of MH being a secondary goal.

9.2 Surgical Technique

The surgical correction will depend on the CT scan findings and symptomatology. The majority of these patients would be candidates for a septoplasty. In fact, of all the intranasal techniques that are available, septoplasty will probably yield the most benefit to the patient, even if the other pathological findings are not eliminated. A properly done septoplasty will take away the rigid wall or spur that is in contact with the turbinates, thus reducing the impact of the contact. However, combining the septoplasty with reduction of turbinate on the contact area offers a higher level of confidence for success.

Surgery is invariably performed under general anesthesia as an outpatient operation. Although topical anesthesia enforced with injection of local anesthetic could be sufficient for minor procedures, it is not an optimal way of dealing with the major intranasal pathology. Under most scenarios, general anesthesia is preferred. The nose is infiltrated with Xylocaine containing 1:100,000 epinephrine along the sidewalls, the dorsum, the roof, and floor of the nose. Topical application using pads saturated with anesthetic and vasoconstrictive agents such as neosynephrine will further reduce the vascularity and intensify the vasoconstrictive effect of the injected materials. The turbinates are injected with Xylocaine containing 1:100,000 epinephrine.

Septoplasty is performed through an L-shaped (Killian) incision. The incision is made on the left side by a right-handed surgeon (▶ Fig. 9.1). The mucoperichondrial flap is elevated on the left side of the septum (▶ Fig. 9.2). The incision is then taken through the septal cartilage only using the sharp end of the septal elevator to avoid penetration of the right side mucoperichondrium (▶ Fig. 9.2). The mucoperichondrium on the right side of the septum is elevated posteriorly, extending to almost the nasopharynx and posterior wall of the nose. The dissection is also continued along the caudal portion of the cartilage and septum, the vomer plate, and perpendicular plate of the ethmoid bone. It is always easier to elevate the posterior portion of the periosteum and extend the dissection anteriorly along the floor on each side of the vomer bone (▶ Fig. 9.3). The septal cartilage incision is then extended to the ethmoid bone (▶ Fig. 9.4). At this level, using the sharp end of the septal elevator, the quadrangle septal cartilage is gently pried away from the perpendicular plate of the ethmoid bone (▶ Fig. 9.5). This dissection is continued posteriorly and caudally at the junction of the vomer bone and the cartilage in a step-by-step fashion until the cartilage is completely free. The cartilage is then removed leaving as much of the straight portion of the septal L frame as possible, a minimum of 20 mm anteriorly and 10 mm caudally (▶ Fig. 9.6). This will expose bony irregularities and spurs to their fullest extent. The deviated portion of the vomer bone and the ethmoid plate are removed using a double-ac-

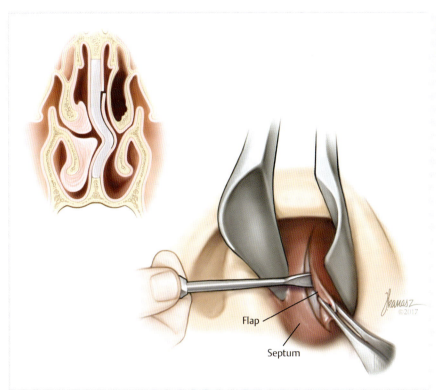

Fig. 9.1 Septoplasty is performed through an **L**-shaped (Killian) incision. The incision is made on the left side for a right-handed surgeon.

Flap

Septum

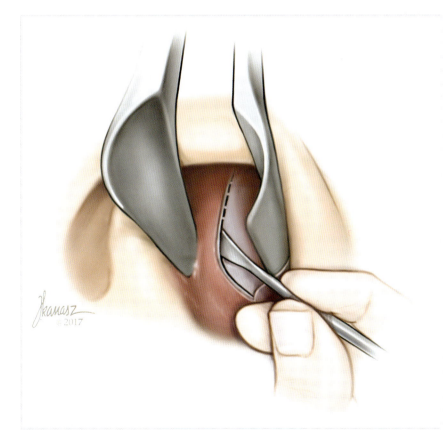

Fig. 9.2 The incision is then taken through the septal cartilage only using the sharp end of the septal elevator to avoid penetration of the right side mucoperichondrium.

tion rongeur (▶ Fig. 9.7). It is crucial to examine both sides of the nasal cavity thoroughly to assure that the spur and the deviated portion of the septum are removed completely. The straight portion of the removed septal cartilage is placed back in position and the mucosa incision is repaired using 5–0 chro-

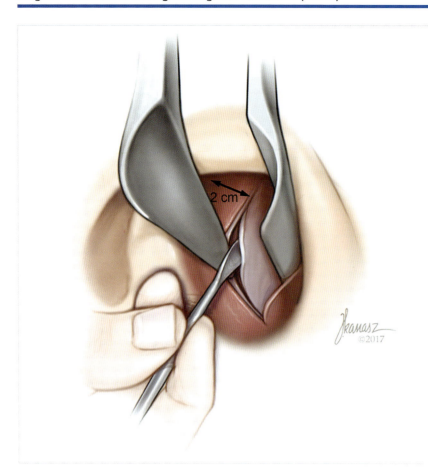

Fig. 9.3 The mucoperichondrium on the right side of the septum is elevated posteriorly, extending to almost the nasopharynx and posterior wall of the nose. The dissection is also continued along the caudal portion of the cartilage and septum, the vomer plate, and perpendicular plate of the ethmoid bone. It is always easier to elevate the posterior portion of the periosteum and extend the dissection anteriorly along the floor on each side of the vomer bone.

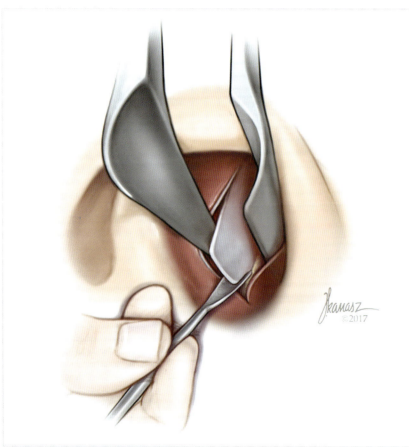

Fig. 9.4 The septal cartilage incision is then extended to the ethmoid bone. At this level, using the sharp end of the septal elevator, the quadrangle septal cartilage is gently pried away from the vomer bone.

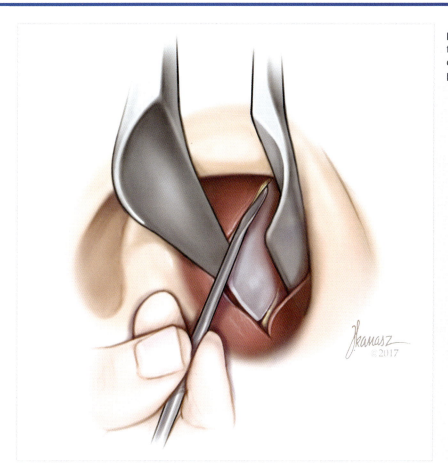

Fig. 9.5 At this level, using the sharp end of the septal elevator, the quadrangle septal cartilage is gently pried away from the perpendicular plate of the ethmoid bone.

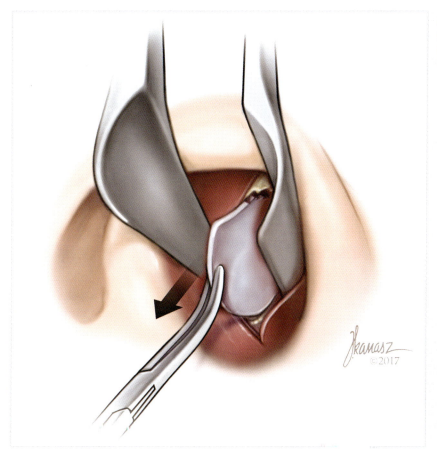

Fig. 9.6 The cartilage is then removed leaving as much of the straight portion of the septal L frame as possible, a minimum of 20 mm anteriorly and 10 mm caudally.

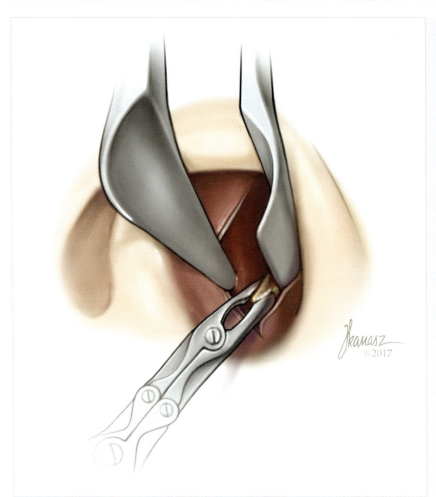

Fig. 9.7 The deviated portion of the vomer bone and the ethmoid plate are removed using a double-action rongeur.

mic running, quilting suture (▶Fig. 9.8; also see ▶Video 9.1). The mucosa incision is repaired using 5–0 chromic running, quilting suture (▶Fig. 9.9).

If the inferior turbinates are enlarged, they can be either outfractured or reduced using turbinate scissors or a number 2 XPS blade (▶Fig. 9.10; see ▶ Video 9.1).

In the presence of septa-bullosa, the bulging portion of the septa-bullosa is also removed, which connects the ethmoid sinus to the space between the two layers of mucoperiosteum. The medial wall of the concha bullosa is removed using a number 4 XPS shaver or with a rongeur (▶Fig. 9.11; see ▶Video 9.1). If the remaining portion of the turbinate becomes unstable, it is removed to avoid blockage of the sinus opening. Excision of the turbinate will be done very conservatively, just enough to eliminate the contact points at the middle and superior turbinate level and a normal size inferior turbinate is left behind. The raw area is then cauterized using suction cautery. If the CT scan confirms the presence of concha bullosa with contact points, the medial wall of the turbinate is removed with a number 4 XPS shaver. This is different from

sinus headache surgery without contact points where the role is to decompress the concha bullosa when the lateral wall of the concha bullosa can be removed to allow better drainage of the sinuses, more physiologic aeration of the sinuses, and elimination of headaches. Haller's cells, if present, can be decompressed by removing the medial wall of the cell. Removal of the caudal portion of the middle turbinates may, by virtue of removing the offending sphenopalatine branches, eliminate the MH. However, turbinectomy should be conservative to avoid any dryness of the nose that can ensue following aggressive removal of the turbinates. Hemostasis is very meticulously secured. The turbinates are often sprayed with thrombin at the end of the operation. The Doyle stents are inserted and fixed in position using 5.0 Prolene sutures and the long ends of the suture are buried inside the Doyle cannula on the left side to minimize irritation of the nasal lining which can produce incessant sneezing. The knot is routinely placed on the left side to facilitate finding the knot during removal of the Doyle stents.

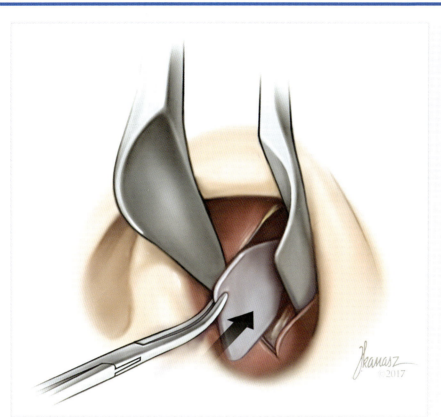

Fig. 9.8 The straight portion of the removed septal cartilage is placed back in position.

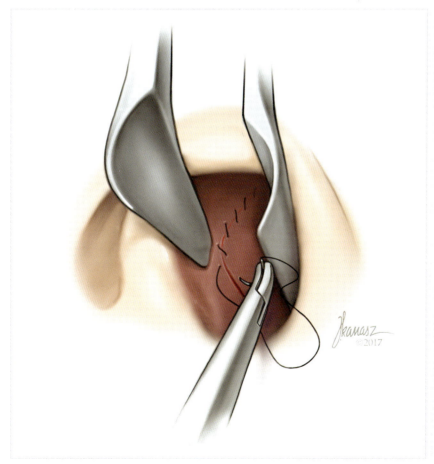

Fig. 9.9 The mucosa incision is repaired using 5–0 chromic running, quilting suture.

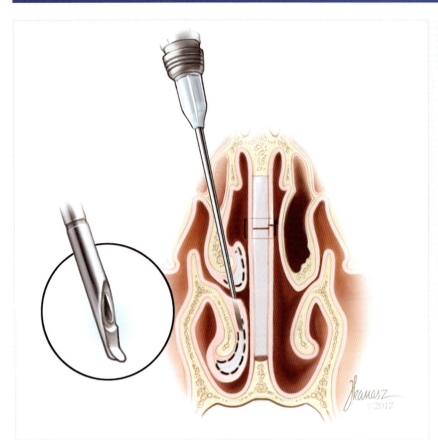

Fig. 9.10 If the inferior turbinates are enlarged, they can be either outfractured or reduced using turbinate scissors or a number 2 XPS blade.

9.3 Postoperative Care

Postoperatively, these patients will have the Doyle stents in place for 4 to 8 days depending on the magnitude of surgery and how far the patient lives. The patient will start nose irrigation using NeilMed solution twice a day as soon as the Doyle stents are removed. The initial irrigations should be very gentle and after the first week or two, the patient will irrigate the nose more vigorously for about 1 month. These patients are kept on antibiotics (Augmentin or ciprofloxacin) for a period of 3 weeks to allow for complete re-epithelialization of the nasal cavity and to reduce the potential for sinus infection. Blowing the nose is avoided for 3 weeks.

The patients are instructed to refrain from strenuous activities for 3 weeks. They are also informed that the surgery at this site may not result in immediate elimination or improvement of MH because of the potential raw area where the nerves could be irritated while healing. Often the positive changes are gradual at this site, unlike some of the other sites where the positive changes are observed either immediately after the surgery or within a short period of time. However, we have had a number of patients who have had MH the night after surgery and no headaches subsequently.

9.4 Complications

One of the potential complications is excessive postoperative bleeding. Most patients will have some bloody drainage, but this is seldom excessive. Use of desmopressin or tranexamic acid in the event of excessive bleeding during surgery or epistaxis postoperatively has been extremely successful in stopping the bleeding without having to pack the nose.[1] In fact, continuous bleeding following removal of the Doyle stents and need for insertion of packing has not been observed in the 18 years that the author has been performing migraine surgery. The dose of desmopressin is 0.3 μg/kg of body weight dissolved in 50 mL of saline, and it is infused over 45 minutes. A potential side effect of the use of desmopressin is hypotension if it is infused too fast. If the patient is volume depleted being on diuretics, one has to carefully monitor blood pressure while the desmopressin is being infused. There is a chance of postoperative reduction in urine volume that should not be alarming. The main contraindication for the infusion of desmopressin is the presence of active coronary artery disease. Tranexamic acid is used in the dose of 10 mg/Kg of body weight through intravenous approach or orally and is repeated every 8 hours if needed.

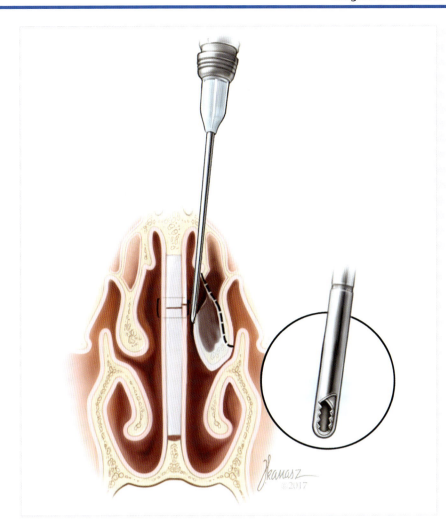

Fig. 9.11 The medial wall of the concha bullosa is removed using a number 4 XPS shaver or with a rongeur.

The other potential complication includes infection. This has been completely eliminated with the 3-week course of antibiotics. An aggressive superior turbinectomy may result in a cerebrospinal fluid leak, which is unlikely. If such a leak is observed, the site is patched with a small piece of nasal lining and packed with Surgicel, and the patient is monitored very closely postoperatively while oral antibiotic is continued.

Septal perforation is another complication of this operation. If a septal tear is observed during the surgery on one side of the mucoperichondrium, while the opposite side is intact, there is no reason for concern. If the tears are bilateral but are at different levels and not apposing, they should heal without persistent perforation. However, if the septal tears are bilateral and these are opposing each other, it is important to replace the straight portion of the removed cartilage or a PDS plate across the perforated area and place a Doyle stent on each side, keeping it in position for at least 8 days and preferably 3 weeks.

If the perforation is discovered weeks or months later and it is less than 1 cm in diameter, through a unilateral transfixion incision, the mucoperichondrium is separated across the perforation and a straight piece of cartilage, fascia, dermis, PDS plate, or Alloderm is placed across the perforation. A simple stent is applied on each side and sutured in place using a through and through Prolene suture, which is removed in 3 weeks.

Patients may not respond favorably to this surgery. Commonly, the reason for the failure of surgery is a conservative approach, which is preferred to the radical removal of the turbinates that could otherwise result in dryness of the nose. Should the patient complain of continuous retrobulbar MH, a CT scan would help to decide whether there are residual contact points, and with that being the case, whether the patients should have additional surgery. However, such decisions should not be reached for 2 to 3 months. Dryness of the nose is extremely rare with conservative surgery. We have not observed an empty nose syndrome following a nose-related migraine surgery.

References

[1] Faber C, Larson K, Amirlak B, Guyuron B. Use of desmopressin for unremitting epistaxis following septorhinoplasty and turbinectomy. Plast Reconstr Surg 2011;128(6):728e–732e

10   Surgical Treatment of Occipital Migraine Headaches (Site IV)

Bahman Guyuron

Salient Points

- Roughly 40% of patients with migraine headaches experience pain in the occipital area.

- Many of these patients have a history of whiplash injury and sometimes the pain is related to occipital neuralgia rather than migraine headaches.

- The headaches related to this site start from the paramedian occipital area where the nerve emerges from the semispinalis muscle (3–3.5 cm caudal to the occipital tuberosity and 1.5 cm from the midline or laterally).

- To detect the occipital trigger site, the patient is asked to point to the migraine headache starting site with a fingertip and a Doppler signal is searched; if present, the site is marked and later tattooed with brilliant green after induction of anesthesia.

- When a Doppler signal is identified, it is usually several centimeters lateral to the site of the emergence of the nerve from the muscle and often where the nerve is intertwined with the occipital artery or its branches.

- With the patient in a sitting position, the midline of the occipital area is identified by palpating the cervical spines and marked.

- With the patient in a supine position, general anesthesia is induced and the patient is turned to the prone position with the shoulders pulled caudally and taped to the bed and the breasts and chest supported with folded rolls.

- Under sterile conditions, an incision is made about 4.5 cm in length at the midline extending from the hairline to the occipital tuberosity after injection of the area with 1% lidocaine containing 1:100,000 epinephrine.

- The skin incision is taken through the trapezius fascia and the muscle, if it extends to the midline, 0.5 to 0.75 cm from the midline on each sided while keeping about a 1–1.5-cm width of the midline raphe intact.

- The trapezius muscle with its oblique fibers may or may not extend to the midline.

- Deep to the trapezius muscle and the underlying fascia, the nerve can be identified with minimal dissection using a pair of Metzenbaum scissors.

- The most common reason for the difficulty in locating the greater occipital nerve is the dissection being conducted superficial to the trapezius muscle instead of the semispinalis capitis muscle.

- If the nerve appears too small, it is likely that there is intramuscular branching and it is crucial to look for additional nerve branches emerging from the muscle.

- As the nerve comes into view, it is isolated with blunt dissection and a vessel loop is passed around it.

- A 2-cm-long block of the muscle between the greater occipital nerve and the midline raphe is isolated and removed using the coagulation power of the cautery.

- A triangular piece of the trapezius fascia and muscle fibers (if present) are then removed laterally overlying the nerve.

- The fascia overlying the nerve is released in a manner similar to carpal tunnel release, the endpoint being visualization of the subcutaneous tissues.

- The vessels commonly surrounding the nerve are isolated and cauterized with a bipolar cautery and transected.

- On patients who have an identifiable Doppler signal, the tattoo marks that were placed earlier are located internally and the vessels are identified and cauterized.

- Should the vessel not be visualized internally in the tattooed area through the main incision, a separate skin incision is made to remove the vessels identified with the Doppler.

- A wedge of muscle is removed lateral to the nerve to accommodate the subcutaneous flap only if the nerve is too medial to have a straighter course without tension if it has to wrap around the medial border of the semispinalis capitis muscle.

- The third occipital nerve is either decompressed or transected as far caudally as possible and allowed to retract in the semispinalis capitis muscle, whenever it is encountered.

- A caudally based subcutaneous flap approximately 2 to 2.5 cm in diameter is elevated cephalad to the course of the nerve and it is placed under the nerve on each side while avoiding constriction of the nerve.

- The flap is attached to the midline with 5–0 Monocryl suture if the procedure is done unilaterally.

- If the procedure is done bilaterally, the suture is passed through one flap and passed under the midline raphe to catch the opposite flap and passed through the midline raphe again and tied to approximate the two flaps to the midline raphe with one stitch as deep as possible.

- The trocar attached to the TLS drain is passed through the subcutaneous tissues and retrieved through the skin above the upper limits of the skin incision, and passed through the midline raphe to drain both sides and is fixed in position using 5–0 plain catgut.

- The deep layer is repaired using an inverted 5–0 Monocryl or Vicryl attaching the subcutaneous tissues to the midline raphe and the skin is repaired using 5–0 plain catgut running locking suture.

- The drain is removed in 3 to 4 days, depending on the amount of the drainage.

10.1 Introduction

Approximately 40% of patients who suffer from migraine headaches (MHs) have occipital MH as a component of their migraine complex. The headaches could be arising from the lesser, greater, and third occipital nerves. In this chapter, we will be focusing on the greater and third occipital nerves related MHs and occipital neuralgia.

Patients who have occipital MH usually have pain starting in the upper neck and occipital region in isolation or in conjunction with MH involving the other sites. Many of these patients have a history of whiplash injury and sometimes the pain is related to occipital neuralgia rather than MH. The latter headaches are often daily with some exacerbation caused by a variety of factors. The patients may point to the mid-occipital area or slightly laterally as the starting sites, while the lesser occipital headaches are usually close to the hairline more laterally.

On examination, many of these patients have tenderness in the site of emergence of the occipital nerve from the semispinalis capitis muscle, which is often 3 to 3.5 cm caudal to the occipital tuberosity and 1.5 cm lateral to the midline. These headaches usually extend cephalically and laterally above the ear. The trapezius and the semispinalis capitis muscles are almost invariably tight and they are commonly very tender. Occasionally, an induration is palpated in the vicinity of the exit point of the nerve from the semispinalis capitis muscle. If the patient can point to a consistent trigger site with a fingertip, the area is marked and explored with a Doppler. Should there be vascular signal, the marking is reinforced.

10.2 Surgical Treatment of Occipital Migraine Headache

In a sitting position, the midline and the lowest portion of the occipital hairline is marked, a small amount of hair is shaved along the incision site and where the vascular signal is identified, and the site is tattooed using brilliant green or methylene blue later when the patient is under anesthesia. An incision is designed about 4 to 5 cm in length at the midline extending from the hairline to the occipital tuberosity (▶Fig. 10.1).

With the patient in a supine position, general anesthesia is induced with endotracheal intubation since the patient will be placed in a prone position and control of an airway can be difficult with laryngeal mask airway. The patient is then turned in a prone position. The shoulders are retracted caudally with 1-inch adhesive tape and the head is supported in a horseshoe head piece. The chest is lifted over the rolls and the breasts are protected in a female patient. The head is prepped and draped. Xylocaine containing 1:100,000 epinephrine is injected at the incision sites and laterally. The 4.5-cm midline incision mark is enforced and the incision is made using a number 10 blade. A self-retainer retractor is placed into position. The incision is deepened to the midline raphe at which level it is directed 0.5 to 0.75 cm laterally (off the midline) on each side leaving 1 to 1.5 cm of the midline raphe intact (▶Fig. 10.2). If the third occipital nerve is encountered and it is larger than 0.15 to 0.2 cm, it is decompressed. However, most of the time, this nerve is very small and runs within the fascia, making the decompression very complicated. In this case, the third occipital nerve is pulled cephalically as much as

possible, transected, and allowed to retract caudally or preferably it is buried in the semispinalis capitis muscle. The fibers of the trapezius muscle, which are oriented obliquely, may extend to the midline in some patients (▶Fig. 10.3). The dissection is continued deeper to the trapezius muscle and fascia until the vertical fibers of the semispinalis capitis muscle are identified. The self-retainer retractor is placed deeper to retract the midline raphe and the incised margin of the trapezius muscle and the fascia, and further lifted with a pair of double hooks. Deep to the trapezius muscle and the underlying fascia, the nerve can be identified with minimal dissection using a pair of Metzenbaum scissors (▶Fig. 10.4). Sometimes the nerve is lateral and requires extra dissection. If there is difficulty in locating the greater occipital nerve, one has to ensure that the dissection is not being conducted superficial to the trapezius muscle, which is the most common reason for the inability to find the nerve during this surgery by the inexperienced operator. Occasionally, this nerve is located very close to the medial border of the muscle. If the nerve appears too small, it is likely that there is intramuscular branching and it is crucial to look for additional nerve branches emerging separately through the muscle. As the nerve comes into view, it is isolated with blunt dissection and a vessel loop is passed around it (▶Fig. 10.5).

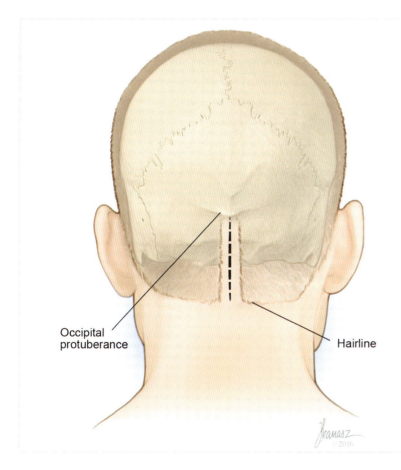

Fig. 10.1 An incision is designed about 4 to 5 cm in length at the midline extending from the hairline to the occipital tuberosity.

Occipital protuberance

Hairline

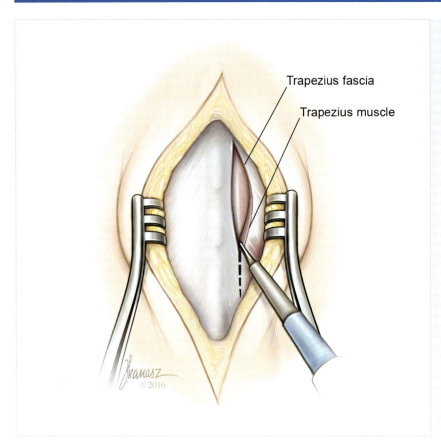

Fig. 10.2 The incision is deepened to the trapezius fascia at which level it is directed 0.5 to 0.75 cm laterally (off the midline) on each side leaving 1 to 1.5 cm of the midline raphe intact.

Trapezius fascia

Trapezius muscle

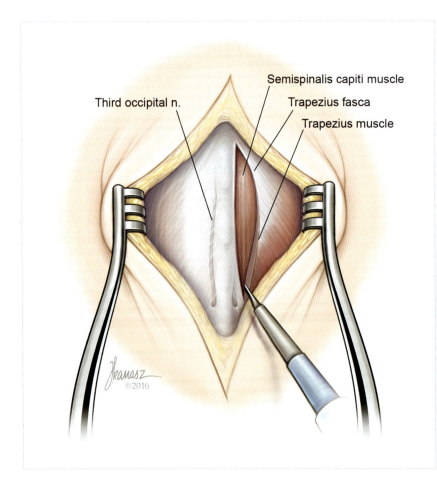

Fig. 10.3 The fibers of the trapezius muscle, which are oriented obliquely, may extend to the midline on some patients.

Semispinalis capiti muscle

Third occipital n.

Trapezius fasca

Trapezius muscle

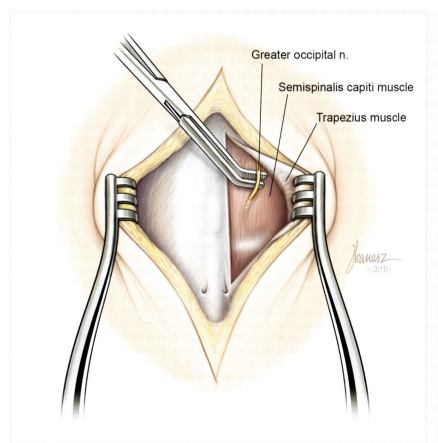

Greater occipital n.

Semispinalis capiti muscle

Trapezius muscle

Fig. 10.4 Deep to the trapezius muscle and the underlying fascia, the nerve can be identified with minimal dissection using a pair of Metzenbaum scissors.

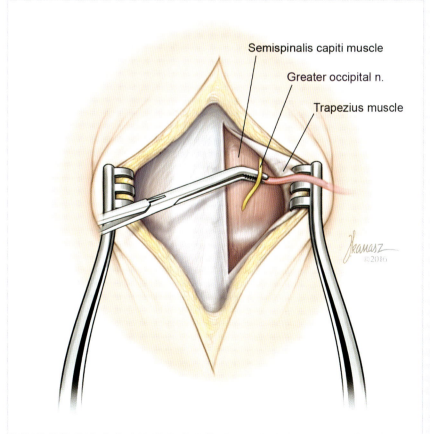

Semispinalis capiti muscle

Greater occipital n.

Trapezius muscle

Fig. 10.5 As the nerve comes into view, it is isolated with fine blunt dissection and a vessel loop is passed around it.

The semispinalis muscle is dissected around the nerve and the segment of the muscle medial to the nerve approximately 2 to 2.5 cm in length is separated from the midline raphe. A munion clamp is placed across the muscle caudal to the nerve and the muscle is transected caudally using the coagulation power of the cautery. Next, the freed block of the muscle is pulled caudally with the munion clamp and transected cephalically, removing this segment of muscle medial to the nerve (▸Fig. 10.6). The nerve is isolated with gentle dissection in the lateral and cephalic direction while the muscle is being removed.

A triangular piece of the trapezius fascia and muscle fibers (if present) is then removed laterally over the nerve (▸Fig. 10.7). The nerve is further isolated with a spreading technique using a fine hemostat. The fascia overlying the nerve is incised with the cautery in a manner similar to carpal tunnel release (▸Fig. 10.8). This is continued laterally to the extent of about 3 to 4 cm. The endpoint is reaching the subcutaneous plane. The occipital artery or its branches that are passing over the nerve, intertwined with it, or travel between the nerve branches are ligated with bipolar cautery and transected (▸Fig. 10.9). On patients who have an iden- tifiable Doppler signal, the preoperatively marked area is tattooed deep prior to the incision and the tattoo material is identified internally leading to the vessels that are similarly dissected and cauterized. Should the vessel not be visualized internally in the tattooed area through the main incision, a separate skin incision is made in the marked area to find and remove the vessels detected with the Doppler.

Rarely, a wedge of the semispinalis capitis muscle is removed lateral to the nerve to accommodate the subcutaneous flap only if the nerve is too medial to take a straight course. This prevents wrapping the nerve around the medial border of the muscle with tension. A caudally based subcutaneous flap approximately 2 to 2.5 cm in diameter is elevated while watching to ensure that the hair follicles are not damaged (▸Fig. 10.10). This flap is designed cephalad to the course of the nerve to allow its placement without constricting the nerve. The nerve is freed enough to be able to advance the subcutaneous flap under it with ease. The subcutaneous flap is passed under the nerve to isolate and shield it from the muscle (▸Fig. 10.11). The flap is attached to the deepest portion of the

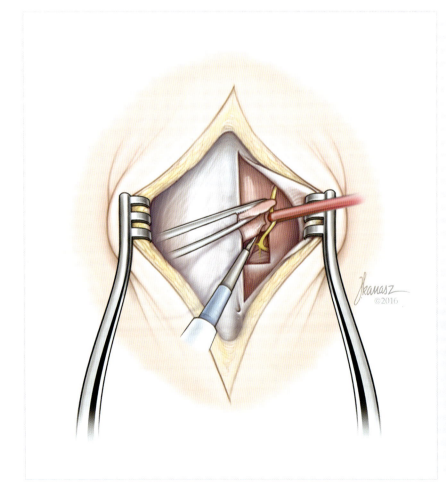

Fig. 10.6 The freed block of the muscle is pulled caudally with the munion clamp and transected cephalically, removing this segment of muscle medial to the nerve.

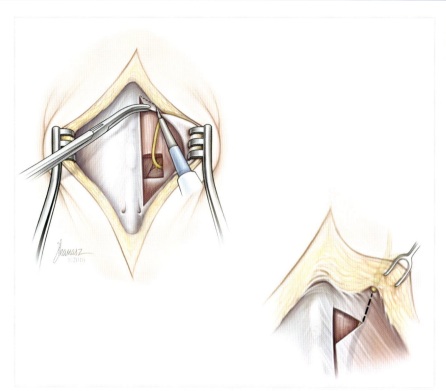

Fig. 10.7 A triangular piece of the trapezius fascia and muscle fibers, if present, is then removed laterally over the nerve.

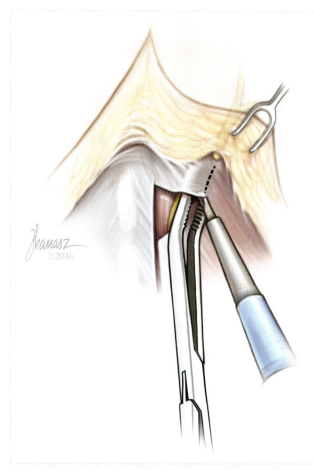

Fig. 10.8 The fascia overlying the nerve is incised with the cautery in a manner like carpal tunnel release.

midline raphe using a 5–0 Monocryl suture, if the procedure is done unilaterally. If the procedure is done bilaterally, the suture is passed through one flap, passed through the deepest portion of the midline raphe to catch the opposite flap, and then passed through the midline raphe again and tied to approximate the two flaps to the midline raphe with one stitch as deep as possible (▶ Fig. 10.12). A TLS drain is brought out through a separate opening using the trocar attached to it, placed in position, and passed through the midline raphe via a minor rent to drain both sides. The drain is fixed in position using 5–0 Prolene immediately after its insertion to avoid any displacement. The deep subcutaneous layer is repaired using inverted 5–0 Monocryl or Vicryl attaching the subcutaneous tissues to the midline raphe to eliminate the dead space (▶ Fig. 10.13), and the skin is repaired using 5–0 plain catgut running locking suture (▶ Fig. 10.14). The incision is covered with bacitracin ointment. The patient is turned in the supine position, extubated, and sent to the recovery room (see ▶ Video 10.1).

10.3 Postoperative Recovery

These patients may have MH the night of surgery, but usually the day after the surgery they are migraine free and seldom have MH postoperatively. However, the response to the surgery varies from patient to patient. The drain is changed every hour

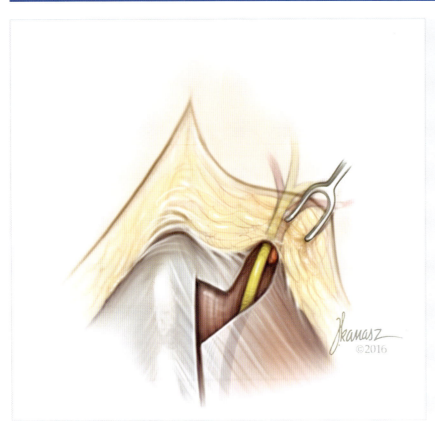

Fig. 10.9 The occipital artery or its branches that are passing over the nerve, intertwined with it or are within the nerve, are ligated with bipolar cautery and transected.

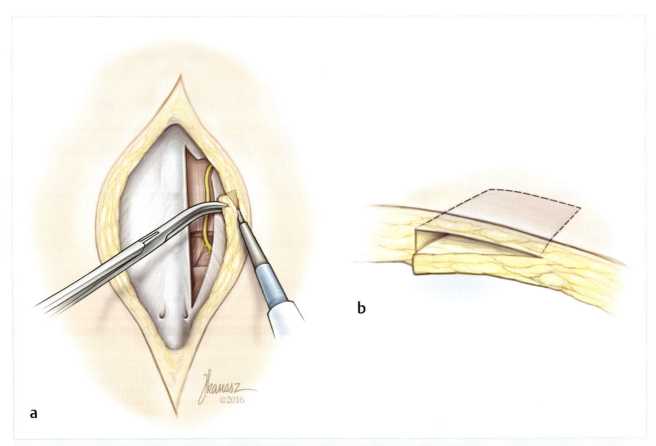

a

b

Fig. 10.10 A caudally based subcutaneous flap approximately 2 to 2.5 cm in diameter is elevated while watching to ensure that the hair follicles are not damaged.

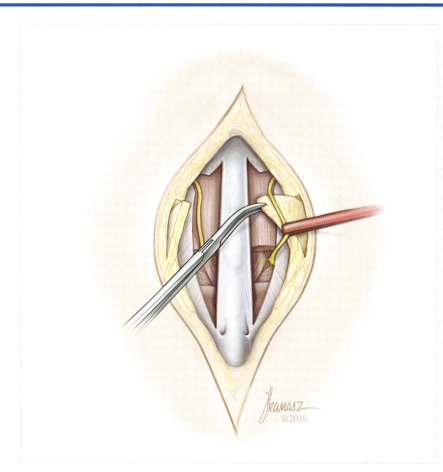

Fig. 10.11 The subcutaneous flap is passed under the nerve to isolate and shield it from the muscle. The flap is attached to the deepest portion of the midline raphe using a 5–0 Monocryl suture, if the procedure is done unilaterally.

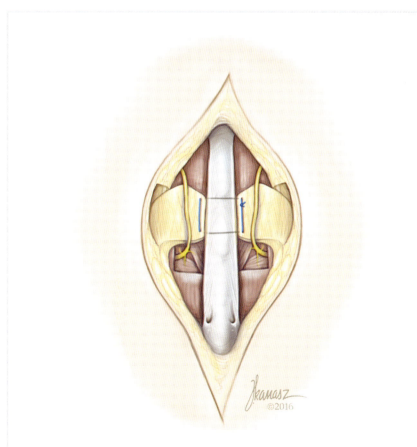

Fig. 10.12 If the procedure is done bilaterally, the suture is passed through one flap, passed through the deepest portion of the midline raphe to catch the opposite flap, and then passed through the midline raphe again and tied to approximate the two flaps to the midline raphe with one stitch as deep as possible.

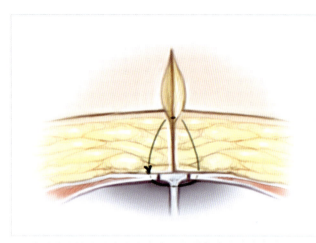

Fig. 10.13 The deep layer is repaired using inverted 5–0 Monocryl or Vicryl attaching the subcutaneous tissues to the midline raphe to eliminate the dead space.

or two the day of surgery, three to four times after that, and removed in 3 to 4 days depending on the magnitude of drainage. The patient is allowed to return to light exercises in 2 weeks and full exercise in 3 weeks. The patient is encouraged to very gently maintain a range of motion of the neck starting the day after surgery.

10.4 Complications

Infection and bleeding can happen after this type of surgery, although they are extremely unlikely. All of the patients experience diffuse and intense numbness along the distribution of the greater and the third occipital nerves, which may last from several weeks to several months. Often, the sensory

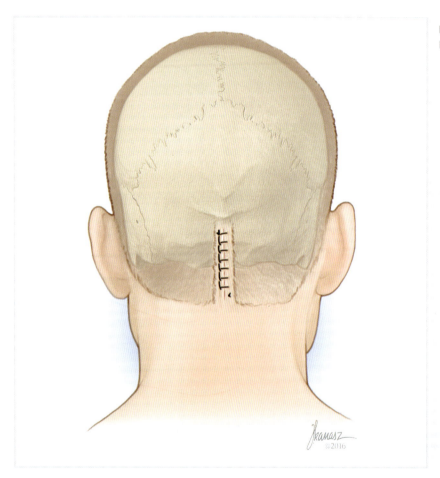

Fig. 10.14 The skin is repaired using 5–0 plain catgut running locking suture.

recovery is complete. There is a remote chance that the numbness may not disappear completely. The surgical failures are usually related to a residual offending vessel or headache in the area of distribution of the lesser or the third occipital nerve. Often, the remaining headaches are localized and subsequent surgeries can be accomplished under local anesthesia and require simple removal of the vessel and decompression or avulsion of the small branches. The persisting headaches following this surgery usually are more cephalad and lateral related to the lesser occipital nerves. Neuromas can occur, but they are extremely rare. If the patient continues to have symptoms at the site after previous surgery, and it is unquestionably related to the greater occipital nerve, the next option would be to inject 3 to 5 mL of fat containing stem cells in the area. This can be repeated if necessary after partial success. The last resort is neurectomy through the same incisional scar. The nerve would be transected and buried in the semispinalis capitis muscle. This would be extremely uncommon.

11 Surgical Treatment of Auriculotemporal Migraine Headaches (Site V)

Bahman Guyuron

Salient Points

- Migraine headaches arising from the temporal region could be triggered from the zygomaticotemporal, auriculotemporal, or zygomaticofacial branches of the trigeminal nerve.

- Some of these migraine headaches arising from the auriculotemporal region can be mistaken for temporomandibular joint disorders.

- An ultrasound Doppler vessel signal is almost always detectable at the most tender site identified by the patient using only one fingertip to identify the discomfort.

- A nerve block commonly results in complete elimination of the migraine headache as long as the patient reports a headache at the time of examination, especially if the block is done soon after the onset of the headache.

- A superficial temporal arterectomy, with or without a neurectomy of the small branch often crossing the nerve, will often result in elimination or significant improvement of the headache.

- For those patients who have multiple tender sites with positive Doppler signal, those with recurrent pain along the distribution of this nerve, or patients with vague temporal migraine headaches within the hair-bearing area, neurectomy of the main auriculotemporal nerve and main superficial temporal artery would be the best choice.

- This trigger site can always be treated under local anesthesia if it is an isolated site or even if it is combined with the lesser occipital or other localized trigger sites and nummular headaches.

- After injection of the area with lidocaine containing 1:100,000 epinephrine, a 6- to 10-mm incision is made over the Doppler signal site, or a 10- to 15-mm incision is made over the base of the sideburn, if the main auriculotemporal nerve and the main superficial temporal artery are the target of the surgery.

- The main superficial temporal artery or the branch of the superficial artery that was detected preoperatively is dissected with a mosquito hemostat and gently cauterized.

- If the main superficial temporal artery is the target of the surgery, it is isolated, ligated, and transected.

- The nerve branches and the vessels entangled with the arterial branches are removed.

- When the main nerve is large enough, it should be buried in the temporalis muscle.

- The incision is closed using 6–0 Monocryl and 6–0 fast-absorbing catgut.

11.1 Introduction

The origin of temporal migraine headaches (MHs) can be confusing since the headaches can arise from the zygomaticotemporal branch of the trigeminal nerve, from the auriculotemporal nerve, from the terminal branches of these two nerves, or—rarely—from a branch of the zygomaticofacial branch of the trigeminal nerve. Many of the new daily and nummular headaches are related to the auriculotemporal nerve. Some of these MHs arising from the auriculotemporal region can be mistaken for temporomandibular joint conditions. In fact, these two conditions can sometimes coexist. Auriculotemporal MHs may cause headaches anywhere in the temporal region, but they are mostly confined to the hair-bearing portion of the temporal region.

A vessel signal is almost always detected at the most tender site, which can be identified by the patient, using his or her fingertip to point to the area.[1] The patient will often complain about pain in the temple area with variable consistency in location and severity. The patient may initially point to the entire temporal area using the whole hand. Yet with further persuasion, the patient can find the most tender spot from which the MH begins using his or her index fingertip. This site is immediately marked and explored with a Doppler ultrasound, and often the signal is identified with minimal effort. Sometimes one has to move the Doppler probe around to locate the signal. Ironically, the signal is only heard in a single spot in spite of the linear nature of the offending artery.

A nerve block commonly results in complete elimination of the MH, should the patient experience a headache at the time of examination. This is especially common if the nerve block is attempted close to the onset of the headaches. A negative response to the nerve block does not necessarily predict a surgical failure, especially at a later stage and on a patient who has sensitization of the entire area. At this stage, the inflammation has spread beyond the target zone, and the central sensitization phase of the migraine cascade could be in effect.

Management of these MHs will be very different than those arising from the zygomaticotemporal branch of the trigeminal nerve. A superficial temporal branch arterectomy with auriculotemporal branch neurectomy often crossing the nerve will usually be successful. Otherwise, for those patients who have multiple tender sites with a positive ultrasound Doppler signal, those with recurrent pain along the distribution of this nerve or patients with vague temporal MH within the hair-bearing area, neurectomy of the main auriculotemporal nerve, and arterectomy of the main superficial temporal would be the best choice. However, since the auriculotemporal nerve branches before it reaches the sideburn, neurectomy of the isolated branch would often be the first choice, especially if the identified signal site is anterior to the hairline.[2]

Additionally, should the patient have residual headaches at this site following a main auriculotemporal neurectomy, it is likely to be related to the branch of this nerve caudal to the sideburn, the zygomaticofacial branch of the trigeminal nerve, or the zygomaticotemporal branch of the trigeminal nerve. Surgery on the site, identified by the patient and confirmed by the ultrasound Doppler, would still benefit this patient.

11.2 Surgical Technique

This trigger site can always be treated under local anesthesia if it is an isolated site or even if it is combined with the lesser occipital site or multiple small localized sites and nummular headaches. However, general anesthesia will be preferred if this site is being operated on in conjunction with sites I (frontal), II (temporal), III (intranasal), or IV (occipital).

For surgical treatment of auriculotemporal nerve–related headaches, a small amount of hair is shaved over the area identified by the patient and confirmed by the Doppler. The area is then prepped and draped. The site is infiltrated with Xylocaine containing 1:100,000 epinephrine. For the main auriculotemporal surgery, a 10- to 15-mm incision is made within the hair-bearing scalp at the base of the sideburn (▶ Fig 11.1).

The dissection is continued deeper with a mosquito hemostat until the auriculotemporal nerve branch and the superficial temporal artery are identified (▶ Fig 11.2). The vessel is isolated to at least a length of 1.5 to 2 cm, ligated, and transected (▶ Fig 11.3). The nerve is then dissected to a sufficient length, usually 1.5 to 2 cm, to allow burying the main nerve in the temporalis muscle if it is large enough (▶ Fig 11.4). A rent is made in the deep temporal fascia (▶ Fig 11.5), a pocket is created within the thickness of the muscle (▶ Fig 11.6), and the transected nerve end is buried in the muscle. To do so, a 5–0 Prolene suture is passed through the muscle (▶ Fig 11.7), starting from the superficial portion of the deep temporal fascia and passed through this muscle and the underlying temporalis muscle, and retrieved through the created pocket in the muscle. The needle is then passed through the nerve, the muscle, and the fascia, this time starting from the inside muscle pocket and retrieved from outside of the muscle (▶ Fig 11.8) and the temporalis fascia. As the suture is tied, it will pull the nerve inside the muscle (▶ Fig 11.9). The ends of the suture are cut slightly long to facilitate finding the nerve, should

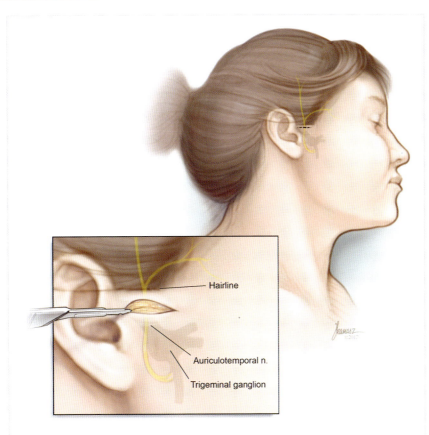

Fig 11.1 A 10- to 15-mm incision is made within the hair-bearing scalp at the base of the sideburn.

Hairline

Auriculotemporal n.

Trigeminal ganglion

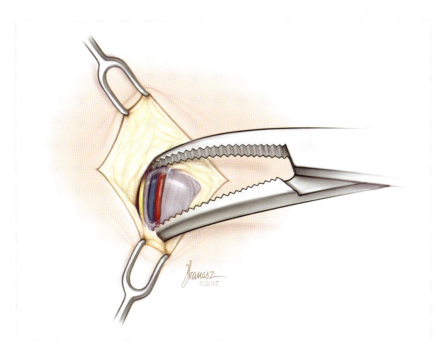

Fig 11.2 The dissection is continued deeper with a mosquito hemostat until the auriculotemporal nerve branch and the superficial temporal artery are identified.

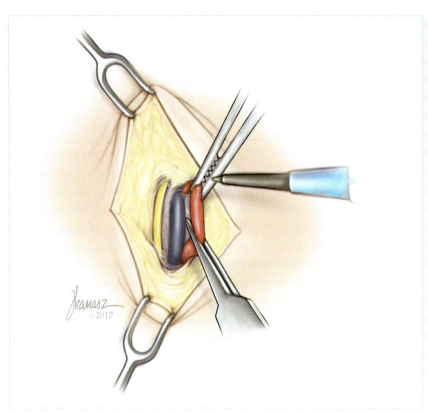

Fig 11.3 The vessel is isolated to at least a length of 1.5 to 2 cm, ligated and transected.

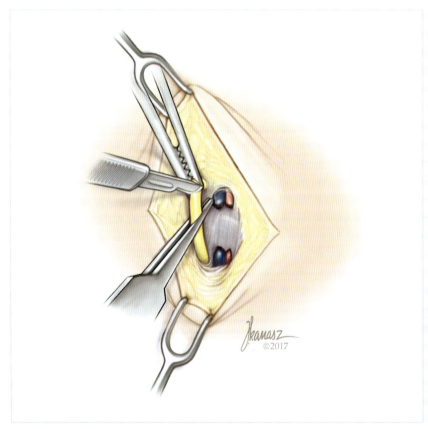

Fig 11.4 The nerve is then dissected to a sufficient length, usually 1.5 to 2 cm, to allow burying the main nerve in the temporalis muscle if it is large enough.

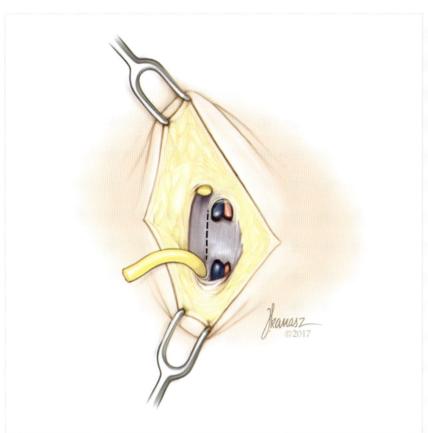

Fig 11.5 A rent is made in the deep temporal fascia.

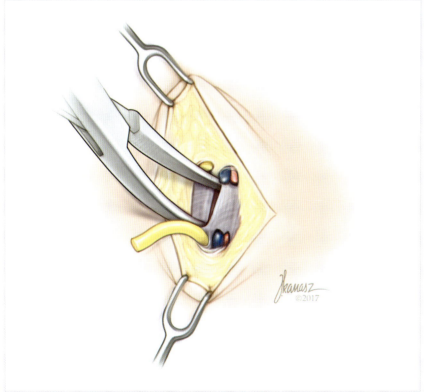

Fig 11.6 A pocket is created within the thickness of the muscle.

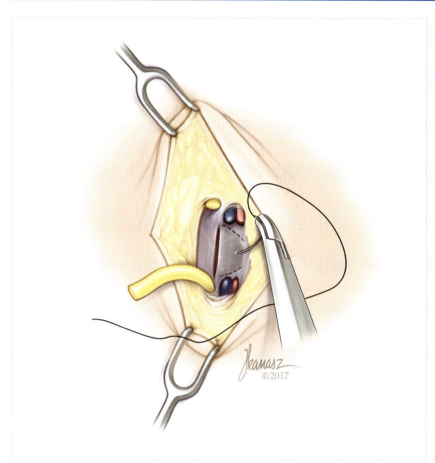

Fig 11.7 A 5–0 Prolene suture is passed through the muscle, starting from the superficial portion of the deep temporal fascia and passed through this muscle and the underlying temporalis muscle, and retrieved through the created pocket in the muscle.

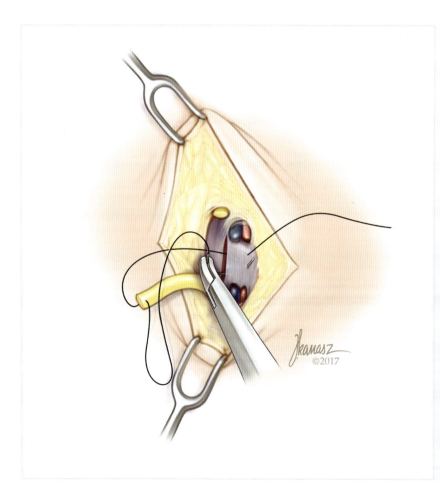

Fig 11.8 The needle is then passed through the nerve, the muscle, and the fascia, this time starting from the inside muscle pocket and retrieved from outside of the muscle and the temporalis fascia.

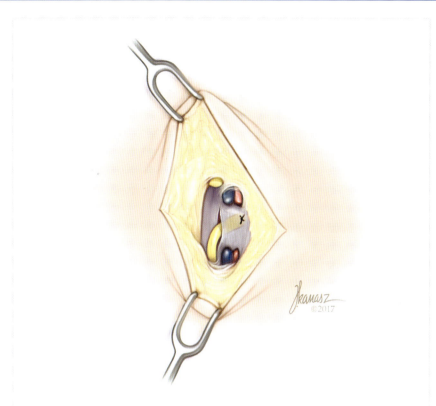

Fig 11.9 As the suture is tied, it will pull the nerve inside the muscle.

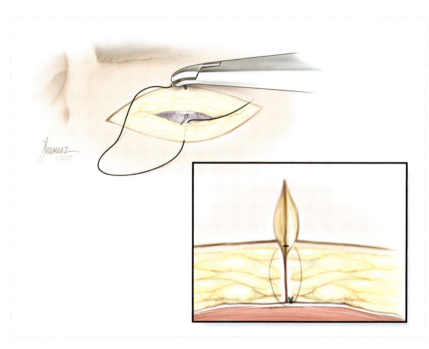

Fig 11.10 The subcutaneous space is eliminated by placing a 6–0 Monocryl suture that would start from the central portion of the incision, catching the deep temporal fascia, passing through the deep portion of the subcutaneous tissue, collecting as much of the deep tissues as possible, retrieved superficially, passed through the opposite superficial layers to the deepest portion of the incision, gathering an equal amount of the tissues and then tied gently to eliminate the dead space and approximate the skin incision margins precisely.

a neuroma be suspected. The subcutaneous space is eliminated by placing a 6–0 Monocryl suture that would start from the central portion of the incision, catching the deep temporal fascia, passing through the deep portion of the subcutaneous tissue, collecting as much of the deep tissues as possible, retrieved superficially, passed through the opposite superficial layers to the deepest portion of the incision, gathering an equal amount of the tissues, and then tied gently to eliminate the dead space and approximate the skin incision margins precisely (▶ Fig 11.10).

The top layer of the skin is repaired using a 6–0 fast-absorbing suture. The incision is covered with Bacitracin ointment.

For any sites other than the main auriculotemporal nerve and the superficial temporal artery, the incision is limited to 6 to 10 mm; the removed vessel length is 5 to 10 mm, and the vessel is dissected and often cauterized or ligated. The nerve branch may or may not be visualized. If the nerve branch is identified, it is only avulsed without burying. The repair technique would be the same as the main auriculotemporal site (see ▶Video 11.1).

11.3 Recovery

These patients can be back to work the same day or the next day, especially if a small branch is the target of the surgery. The patients can resume all normal activities the next day. The repaired incision is covered with Bacitracin ointment twice a day for a week.

11.4 Complications

Wound infection is extremely rare. Hematoma can occur, but since there is no space left for blood collection, we have not observed this. No patient has had a recurrence of pain at exactly the same site. On rare occasions, the patient may observe headaches at different branches of the same nerve, in which case the procedure can be repeated.

References

[1] Guyuron B, Riazi H, Long T, Wirtz E. Use of a Doppler signal to confirm migraine headache trigger sites. Plast Reconstr Surg 2015;135(4):1109–1112
[2] Chim H, Okada HC, Brown MS, et al. The auriculotemporal nerve in etiology of migraine headaches: compression points and anatomical variations. Plast Reconstr Surg 2012;130(2):336–341

12 Surgical Treatment of Lesser Occipital Migraine Headaches (Site VI)

Bahman Guyuron

Salient Points

- The lesser occipital trigger site is the most anatomically unpredictable site.
- A Doppler vascular signal can often be identified in the headache-onset site.
- A nerve block can only be reliable if the patient is experiencing headache at the time of office visit.
- A negative nerve block does not rule out the presence of a lesser occipital trigger site.
- This site is more caudal and lateral to the greater occipital trigger site and it is close to the lateral occipital hairline.
- The surgery is often done under local anesthesia unless some other sites are being decompressed at the same time, mandating the use of general anesthesia.
- A horizontal incision about 1.5–2 cm in length is used to find the nerve and the vessel.
- A fine (mosquito) hemostat is used to continue the dissection with a spreading technique.
- The vessel is dissected to an extent of 1 to 2 cm and cauterized or ligated and excised.
- A nerve decompression or neurectomy could be selected for deactivation of this trigger site.
- If a neurectomy is preferred, the nerve end is buried in the adjacent muscle to reduce the potential for a neuroma formation.
- The patient can return to work the same day or the next day if the dissection is not extensive.

12.1 Introduction

The lesser occipital trigger site is the most problematic of all the migraine sites when it comes to locating the nerve. This is due to the tremendous variation in the anatomy and presentation of the headache site as well as branching pattern of this nerve.[1] Any headache lateral and caudal to the greater occipital nerve territory is likely to be related to the lesser occipital nerve. Commonly, a Doppler vascular signal can be identified at the trigger site. A positive nerve block could prove very informative only if the patient experiences a migraine headache (MH) at the time of the examination. However, when the pain is chronic in nature, the block may not result in cessation of the MH.

12.2 Surgical Technique

With the patient in a sitting position, the most tender spot is identified by the patient and is marked. Ultrasound Doppler vascular signal is searched for to confirm the presence of a vessel. Additionally, the headaches site is confirmed with the patient in a supine position and the head tilted to the side. These two sites in the sitting and supine positions may not always match. One may have to repeat the examination a few times before designing the incision.

A horizontal incision about 1.5 to 2 cm in length is designed and about 1 cm of the surrounding hair is shaved on each side of the incision (▶ Fig. 12.1; see ▶ Video 12.1). The area is infiltrated with Xylocaine containing 1:100,000 epinephrine. If the patient is having MH at the time of surgery, the patient is queried about the level of the pain before and after the injection. While complete disappearance of the pain is often experienced, not having thorough elimination of the MH after injection of the local anesthesia is not prohibitive of surgery. The incision is made and taken down as deep as possible in the subcutaneous plane. A fine (mosquito) hemostat is used to continue the dissection with a spreading technique (▶ Fig. 12.2). Immediately below the trapezius fascia, the nerve, the vessel, or both

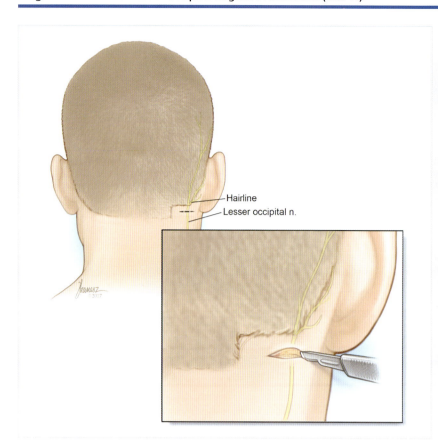

Fig 12.1 A horizontal incision about 1.5 to 2 cm in length is designed and about 1 cm of the surrounding hair is shaved on each side of the incision (Video 12.1).

Hairline

Lesser occipital n.

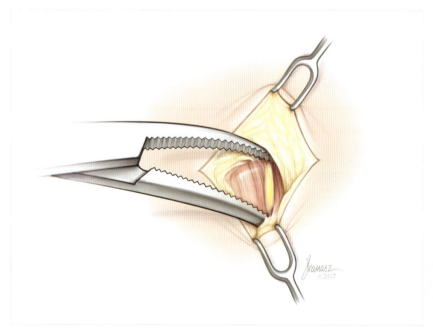

Fig 12.2 A fine (mosquito) hemostat is used to continue the dissection with a spreading technique.

are identified and a rubber band is placed around the nerve (▶ Fig. 12.3). The vessel is dissected to an extent of 1 to 2 cm and cauterized (▶ Fig. 12.4). If a compression site is identified, the fascia is released. However, in most instances, finding a distinct compression site is unlikely. If the exploration fails to detect a compres-

sion site, the nerve is isolated, dissected, and transected to a length of approximately 1.5 cm (▶ Fig. 12.5). A pocket is created in the adjacent trapezius muscle large enough to accommodate the nerve (▶ Figs. 12.6, 12.7). A 5–0 blue Prolene suture is passed through the muscle, retrieved through the created tunnel, then passed

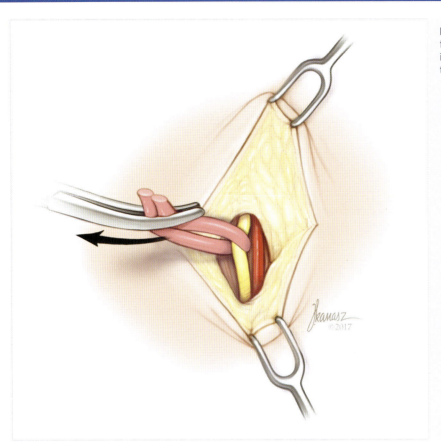

Fig 12.3 Immediately below the trapezius fascia, the nerve, vessel, or both are identified and a rubber band is place around the nerve.

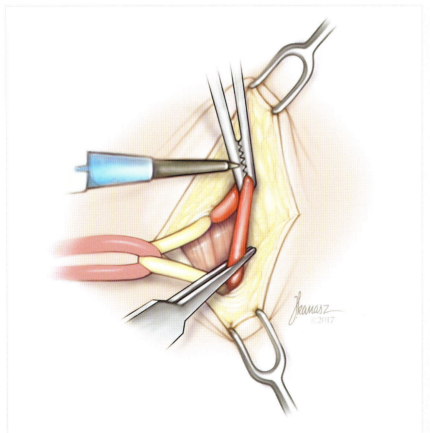

Fig 12.4 The vessel is dissected to an extent of 1 to 2 cm and cauterized.

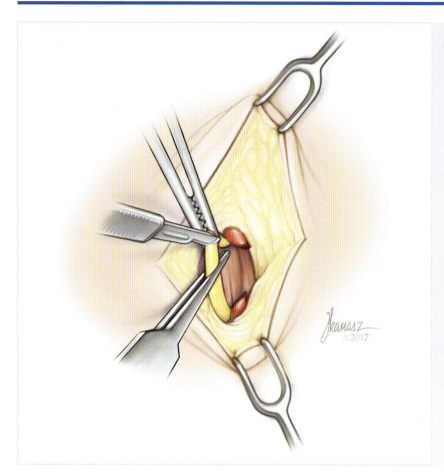

Fig 12.5 If the exploration fails to detect a compression site, the nerve is isolated and dissected and transected to a length of approximately 1.5 cm.

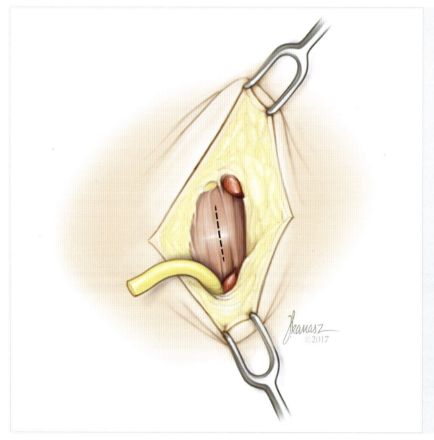

Fig 12.6 A pocket is designed in the adjacent trapezius muscle large enough to accommodate the nerve.

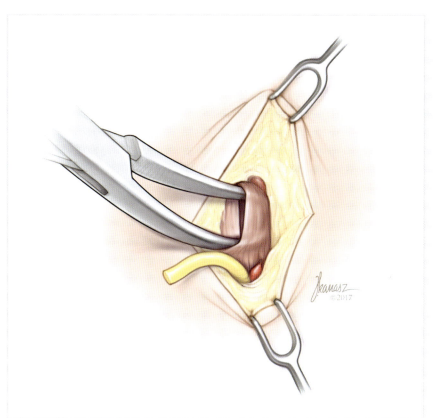

Fig 12.7 The pocket is created using a fine hemostat.

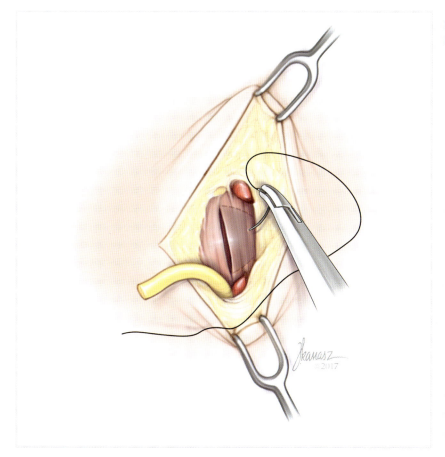

Fig 12.8 A 5–0 blue Prolene suture is passed through the muscle.

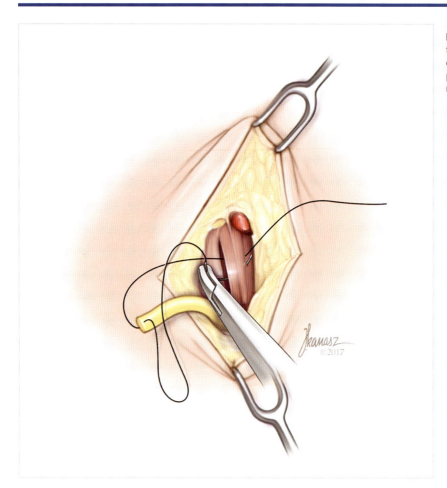

Fig 12.9 The needle is retrieved through the created tunnel, passed through the end of the nerve, brought back through the pocket and the muscle, and tied over the muscle.

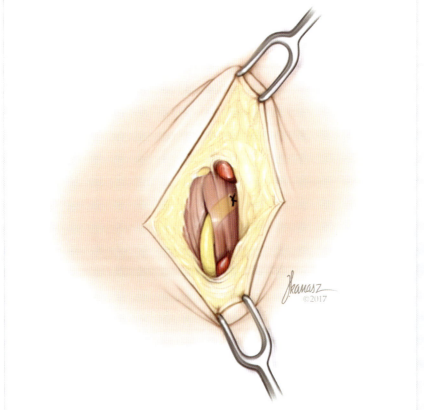

Fig 12.10 As the suture is tied, the nerve end is watched to be pulled into the muscle pocket.

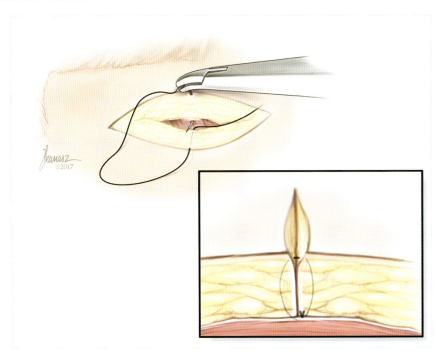

Fig 12.11 A 5–0 Monocryl suture is passed through the deeper layers while catching the base of the dissected area and deeper portion of the subcutaneous tissues, and then through the superficial portion of the subcutaneous tissues and tied to eliminate the dead space.

through the end of the nerve (▶Fig. 12.8), brought back through the pocket and the muscle, and tied over the muscle (▶Fig. 12.9). As the suture is tied, the nerve end is watched to be pulled into the muscle pocket (▶Fig. 12.10). Minute amount of 0.1- to 0.2-mL Kenalog (40 mg/mL) is injected in the area around the nerve end. A 5–0 Monocryl suture is then passed through the deeper layers while catching the base of the dissected area and deeper portion of the subcutaneous tissues, and then through the superficial portion of the subcutaneous tissues and tied to eliminate the dead space (▶Fig. 12.11). The superficial portion of the skin is repaired using a 5–0 plain catgut. The wound is covered with Bacitracin ointment.

12.3 Recovery

Depending on the magnitude of the dissection, most patients could return to work the same or the next day. They are, however, asked to avoid aspirin or NSAIDs (nonsteroidal anti-inflammatory drugs)

and refrain from heavy exercises for 1 week. The wound is covered with Bacitracin ointment for 1 week. The patient is asked to avoid using a hair dryer for a week and to do so with caution for another 2 weeks thereafter.

12.4 Complications

Infection or hematoma is exceedingly rare. There is a potential for emergence of another headache trigger site adjacent to the scar due to frequent arbitration of the nerve. A neuroma can develop at the neurectomy site, but is very unlikely. Alopecia is also a rare possibility.

Reference

[1] Lee M, Brown M, Chepla K, et al. An anatomical study of the lesser occipital nerve and its potential compression points: implications for surgical treatment of migraine headaches. Plast Reconstr Surg 2013;132(6):1551–1556

13 Surgical Treatment of Nummular Headaches (Site VII)

Bahman Guyuron

Salient Points

- Nummular headache (NH) is a disorder in which pain is localized to a specific area.
- NH is a rare disorder occurring with an estimated incidence of 6.4 to 9/100,000 in a hospital-based series.
- ICHD-3 beta describes NH as a sharply contoured pain of highly variable duration, but often chronic, in a small circumscribed area (1–6 cm) of the scalp.
- The pain is often in a round or elliptical-shaped area. It typically occurs in the parietal region and tends to be "side locked."
- The patient can usually point to a distinct and constant spot.
- An ultrasound vascular Doppler signal can almost invariably be detected.
- A positive response to a nerve block could be extremely informative so long as the patients report headaches at the time of office visit.
- Surgery is performed under local anesthesia and involves a 5- to 10-mm incision and removal of a small vessel with or without removal of a terminal nerve branch.
- The incision is repaired with 6–0 Monocryl and 5–0 or 6–0 plain catgut depending on the site.
- Surgery almost uniformly results in elimination of headaches in the operated site.
- There is a small chance of NH developing in the vicinity of the previous surgery site, but never exactly in the same area.

13.1 Introduction

Nummular headache (NH) is a rare disorder occurring with an estimated incidence of 6.4 to 9/100,000 in a hospital-based series,[1,2] nevertheless, this entity seems more common post-migraine surgery than statistics suggest. The International Classification of Headache Disorders, third edition, beta version (ICHD-3 beta) describes NH as a sharply contoured pain of highly variable duration, but often chronic, in a small circumscribed area of the scalp. The pain is often in a round or an elliptical-shaped area. While it typically occurs in the parietal region, it can be anywhere on the scalp. Over-the-counter analgesics are commonly adequate to treat most NH patients. Sometimes the pain is severe, necessitating additional modalities.[3,4]

13.2 Detection of the Trigger Site

The patient is asked to point to the trigger site, and the area is marked. Almost invariably, a vascular signal can be detected with ultrasound Doppler. Occasionally, it is necessary to move the Doppler probe around a few millimeters outside of where the patient points to find the signal. The signal site is then marked. Should the patient report headache at the time of the office visit, the Doppler signal site is injected with 0.5 mL of Naropin. A positive response to a nerve block could be extremely informative as long as the patient reports having a headache at the time of the office visit. A negative nerve block does not mean that surgery will not be effective in the injected site.

13.3 Surgical Procedure

The procedure is done under local anesthesia as an office procedure in the majority of the patients. After the surgical site is identified, the marked area of pain and associated Doppler signal are injected using lidocaine 1% with epinephrine (1:100,000). A 5- to 10-mm incision is designed in the previously marked area. Usually, a 0.5-inch 30-gauge needle is used to inject slowly and with single skin penetration. After awaiting an appropriate time to maximize the anesthetic and vasoconstrictive effect of the injection, a number 15 blade is used to make an incision through the skin and dermis (▶Fig. 13.1). A mosquito hemostat is used for the dissection (▶Fig. 13.2). The direction of the dissection is based on the logical anatomic course of the artery and the nerve in that area. Once the artery is identified, it is dissected both proximally and distally to obtain a segment for removal (▶Fig. 13.3). Larger arteries will require suture ligation using a 5–0 or 6–0 Monocryl, while smaller arteries are adequately treated using targeted cauterization. The entire intervening segment of the artery is removed. Small nerves that are intimately associated with the artery are removed (▶Fig. 13.4) when detected. Larger nerves require division with the cut end buried in the muscle to minimize the potential for a neuroma formation, if a muscle is present in the vicinity of the nerve. After hemostasis is verified, and following assurance that there are no addition-al branches of the nerve or the artery, the incision is closed. The first stitch includes a bite of the deeper tissues to obliterate the dead space. In the hair-bearing areas, a 5–0 plain catgut suture is used, while in exposed areas, a 6–0 fast-absorbing catgut should be employed (▶Fig. 13.5) (see ▶Video 13.1). The incision in sites without hair is covered with waterproof dressing, which is removed in 7 to 8 days. Bacitracin ointment is used where the presence of hair can make adherence of the occlusive dressing difficult.

13.4 Recovery

An antibiotic ointment is applied to the incision site two times a day for 7 days in the absence of waterproof dressing. Patients can shower and gently cleanse the area after 24 to 48 hours. The patients are permitted to return to work and normal activity the same day or the day after the procedure. Narcotic medications are rarely necessary. Infrequently, patients may experience an acute worsening of their headaches the night following the procedure, but this is often self-limiting.

13.5 Complications

Since the procedure is so minor, it harbors minimal risks. Infection would be extremely rare in

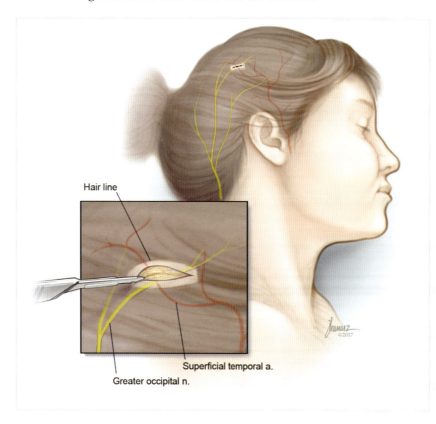

Fig. 13.1 A number 15 blade is used to make an incision through the skin and dermis.

Hair line

Superficial temporal a.

Greater occipital n.

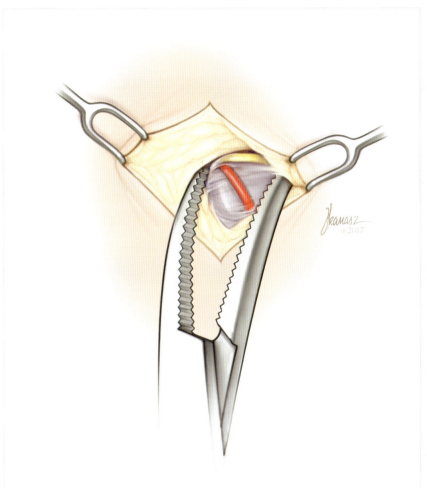

Fig. 13.2 A mosquito hemostat is used for the dissection.

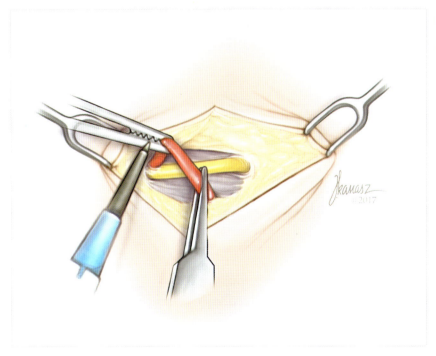

Fig. 13.3 Once the artery is identified, it is dissected both proximally and distally to obtain a segment for removal.

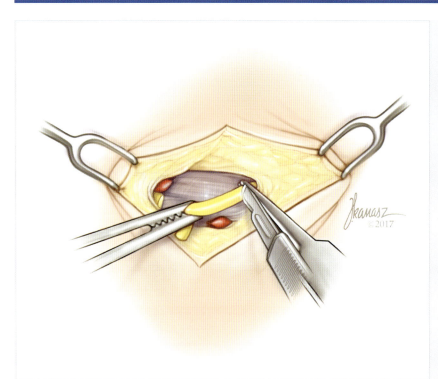

Fig. 13.4 Small nerves that are intimately associated with the artery are removed when detected. Larger nerves require division with the cut end buried in the muscle to minimize the potential for a neuroma formation, if a muscle is present in the vicinity of the nerve.

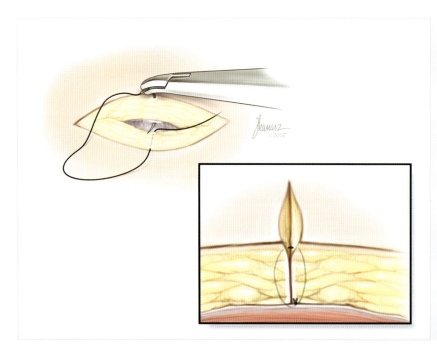

Fig. 13.5 The first stitch with 6-0 Monocryl includes a bite of the deeper tissues to obliterate the dead space. In the hair-bearing areas, a 5–0 plain gut suture is used, while none hair bearing areas 6-0 fast absorbing cat-gut is uses.

these sites. On rare occasions, patients may observe emergence of a new site near the operated scar, but it is almost never exactly in the same area. While formation of a neuroma is a theoretical possibility, it has not been observed at this point.

References

[1] Pareja JA, Pareja J, Barriga FJ, et al. Nummular headache: a prospective series of 14 new cases. Headache 2004;44(6):611–614

[2] Grosberg BM, Solomon S, Lipton RB. Nummular headache. Curr Pain Headache Rep 2007;11(4):310–312

[3] Pareja JA, Montojo T, Alvarez M. Nummular headache update. Curr Neurol Neurosci Rep 2012; 12(2):118–124

[4] Guyuron B, Gatherwright J, Reed D, Ansari H, Knackstedt R.Treatment of Dopplerable nummular headache with and without migraines using auriculotemporal decompression and arterectomy

Index

Note: Page references followed by *f* or *t* indicate material in figures or tables, respectively.

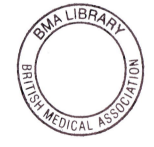

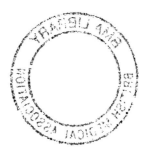